CANDIDA
made simple
♦♦♦

Cheryl Townsley

LFH Publishing
6520 South Broadway, Littleton, CO 80121

Graphics: Nick Zellinger
Text Design: Theresa Frank

This publication is designed to provide accurate and
authoritative information in regard to the subject matter
covered. It is sold with the understanding that the author
and the publisher are not engaged in rendering legal,
medical, or other professional service. If medical services or other expert consultation is required, the services
of a competent professional should be sought.

Townsley, Cheryl
        Candida made simple /
     Cheryl Townsley
        Includes bibliographical references
        ISBN 0-9644566-8-0
        1. Toxicology. 2. Health. 3. Nutrition. I. Title.

For information contact:

LFH Publishing
6520 South Broadway
Littleton, CO 80121
303-794-4477
For ordering information, refer to the last page.

Printed in the United States of America

CONTENTS
✦✦✦

You surely know that your body is a temple

where the Holy Spirit lives.

The Spirit is in you and is a gift from God.

You are no longer your own.

God paid a great price for you.

So use your body to honor God.

1 Corinthians 6: 19 – 20

ACKNOWLEDGMENTS
✦✦✦

As I sat and contemplated this new book, I decided to look up the definition of an author. According to Webster's, an author is "one who makes or creates something." Since I am not God, what I create is made from something else or learned from someone else. It is those "somethings" and "someones" I want to acknowledge. For truly, I have only added my perspective and experience to this vast reservoir of knowledge.

The past several years of practicing health at Lifestyle for Health have brought me in touch with thousands of clients. Whether by phone or office visit, these wonderful people have given me the opportunity to pursue health and effective answers as never before.

Now each set of symptoms has a name and a face. I'm no longer amassing fascinating information, I'm determined to help another human being experience a health breakthrough. Health is truly my ministry, my mission and my call. Thank you each and every client! May you each be blessed with the whole health God has always desired you to have!

The Lifestyle for Health Team has encouraged me to pursue my destiny when I seriously considered stopping. When the load of helping others find health becomes heavy, it is crucial to have friends who will stand in the gap through prayer, friendship and support. For each member of our LFH Team I say "thank you!" May you be blessed with God's best as you also take the message of health to our nation!

Forest and Anna continue to be my most precious supporters. Why pursue health if, in the process, you lose everything important? We have and are continuing to learn how to pursue our destiny and stay in balance as a family. Thank you for teaching me how to laugh, how to have fun and how to share who I am without rejection. I love you both dearly.

A purpose and a destiny are impossible to define if you do not know the God who created you. I thank God He is real in my life. It is my relationship with Him that has helped me unveil my destiny. His is my source of inspiration and wisdom to pursue that destiny with honor. Father, thank you for living in me, loving me and encouraging me to be the person You created me to be!

INTRODUCTION
✦✦✦

I had worked with John (not his real name) and his family. His wife and children were doing well but John had not lost any weight. He was 25+ pounds overweight. I had done my best with nutrition and biofeedback testing. Yet, the weight wouldn't budge. While visiting a health food store, he took a Candida self-test and found he had Candida.

One month and 25 pounds less, John was excited. He came and shared his success with me. I began to study, research and apply my knowledge on myself, my family and my clients. The results were exciting. John's Candida cleanse and protocol became a part of my program and will be shared in this book.

John's success and his willingness to share it with me began a journey that has helped more people than I can count. TV and radio response has indicated the public's desire for information on Candida that is practical, effective and affordable.

In writing each of my books, I have sought to provide information that is practical and affordable. Knowledge that is difficult to understand and/or apply is worse than worthless ... it gives rise to hopelessness. Anyone experiencing the symptoms of Candida does not need the extra burden of wrestling with despair.

Join the millions who are taking back control of their health. In this book, you will be equipped with a foundational understanding of the immune and lymphatic system, while you also learn to identify the vast array of Candida symptoms and the effective weapons to eradicate this menace.

Candida can impact babies, children, men and women. It is no respecter of persons. It hits hard and persistently hangs around. It can also be stopped. You determine who wins — Candida or you. I vote for you ... for you have the weapon in your hand. Read it, use it and build a *lifestyle for health!*

Cheryl Townsley

ONE
BEFORE CANDIDA...
THE IMMUNE SYSTEM
✦✦✦

Many individuals have taken our Living WHOLE Optimal Health program. The majority have experienced improvement in overall health and energy levels. One of the goals of Living WHOLE has also been to help people balance weight — whether they are over weight or under weight. When I found that some people were not losing weight, I began to seek the root of this problem.

How could people feel better, lose many symptoms of sickness and yet still not lose weight? This mystery drove me to deeper research, more in-depth testing with our biofeedback machine and expanded client histories. Within months we stumbled onto a common problem ... Candidiasis.

The more I investigated this yeast-like fungus, the more I found it impacted many of the clients and customers of Lifestyle for Health. In order to help these people, I knew we needed to get to the root of the problem as well as the possible alternatives to address the symptoms.

The real key to understanding how to fight Candidiasis is to understand the role of the immune system. The entire purpose and mission of the immune system is to defend the body against invaders. Whether those invaders are germs, cancer cells, fungi, parasites or other "critters," the immune system is our primary defense system to keep everything in balance.

Although the immune system is quite a complex, miraculous system, its basic strategy is

♦ recognize the enemy
♦ mobilize the military
♦ attack!

When the immune system is unable to recognize, mobilize and/or attack, then the invaders overcome and the person displays sickness in some form. In my study of the immune system, I have become aware of how closely and intimately the lymphatic system interacts with immune functioning. It is virtually impossible to improve the health of the immune system without including the lymphatic system and vice versa.

In order to successfully beat Candidiasis or any sickness, we must have a basic understanding of the immune and lymphatic systems. These two systems are so interrelated that it is impossible to appreciate the significance of one without understanding the other.

Although the following section is somewhat technical, I believe that this overview will underscore the importance of lymphatic support and increased cell communication support in order for any true progress to be made in dealing with immune imbalances, such as Candidiasis.

IMMUNE SYSTEM PROBLEMS

Over the past fifteen years, Dr. Darryl See, a leading immunologist, has discovered that the immune system has decreased in its function by 25% based on N K (Natural Killer) cell function. It is now estimated that the immune system function is dropping at the rate of 3% to 4% each year.[1]

What does that mean to you?

Your ability to fight sickness is decreasing each year and you already have a 25% handicap. Your immune system is your defense system to fight sickness and disease. If you do nothing then your fate is sealed; you ... and your children ... will experience sickness and disease at more and more alarming rates!

Whether your issue is Candidiasis or some other malady, you can benefit by understanding the immune system. Though you may not be educated on this powerful system, your body is more than aware of its importance. Your ignorance only feeds the thieves who are out to steal, kill and destroy your health.

If you are currently facing a heavy load of "brain fog" or are overwhelmed with Candida, you might want to skip this first chapter until you are in a better condition to understand it. Chapters Two through Six will give you the game plan to successfully fight Candida. The entire purpose of this chapter is to give you an understandable overview of the complexity of the immune system. Without a balanced immune system, a person will never keep Candida under control or develop optimal health.

A weakened immune system is the result of several stressers. Let's review these stressers that can undermine any immune system. For more information, please refer to my books *Food Smart!* and *Cleansing Made Simple.*

IMMUNE SYSTEM STRESSERS
STRESSER 1 – DIETARY ROAD BLOCKS
High intake of the bad fats
Many people today are cutting out fat in order to improve their health. Unfortunately they are under the misconception that all fats are the same and all fats are bad. Nothing could be further from the truth. It is true that bad fats are unhealthy; however, there are good fats that are crucial for optimal health.

The American public eats too much of the bad fats and too little of the good fats. The bad fats include animal fats (saturated fats), especially when those animals have been given a diet high in antibiotics, steroids and hormones. If you choose to eat meat, then I highly recommend that you get it from organic, natural sources.

In addition to animal fats, the bad fats include trans fats and hydrogenated fats. These fats are identified on labels with the words *hydrogenated* or *partially hydrogenated*. This type of fat is virtually impossible to assimilate unless it is heated to over 300 degrees. That usually doesn't happen unless you are being cremated!

When cutting out bad fats, do not cut out the good fats. An example of the good fats is essential fatty acids (EFAs) which are a key contributor to building the immune system, the brain, hormones and fluid balancing. No Candida program can be totally successful without the addition of EFAs.[2]

Too many refined carbohydrates — sugar and white flour
The average American consumes over 150 pounds of sugar per year compared to 12 pounds consumed in the early 1800s. It is estimated that one tablespoon of sugar can suppress the immune system by up to 50% for three to four hours. Obviously 150 pounds of sugar plays a big role in compromised immune function.[3]

As important as carbohydrates are in our bodies, those carbs must come primarily from complex sources — vegetables and fruits. Rather than complex carbohydrates, most Americans consume high levels of simple carbohydrates from sources such as white flour pasta, white flour breads, bagels, chips, cookies and other desserts. White flour is believed to impact the body in a similar manner to that of refined sugar. Both hamper immune system function.

Low fiber
A diet comprised of simple carbohydrates and fats rarely contains enough fiber. Fiber is essential for healthy bowel flora, healthy bowel movements and the destruction of Candida.

Fiber comes from roughage which comes from whole grains, fresh fruits and vegetables. Following the recommended Candida diet will automatically increase fiber consumption. Additional fiber is often needed to remedy past deficiencies.

Empty calories from non-nutritious food
In the pursuit of easy weight loss, the average American has sought products that are *low fat*. Many of these products are indeed *low fat*

but contain higher amounts of sugar and are virtually void of any nutrition.

When a person primarily purchases "boxes" at the grocery store, she is buying little coffins of dead stuff. Rarely does the box contain nutrition. She is buying death on the installment plan and is certainly not getting calories from nutritious food. Good nutrition requires daily intake of foods that contain life — primarily fresh, organic, vine-ripened fruit, vegetables and whole grains.

Food additives, preservatives and food dyes
The healthier I get, the more I come to recognize the negative impact of additives, preservatives and food dyes. Foods containing those stressers immediately produce symptoms in my body that are not pleasant. This is true not only of me but of most people. Unfortunately, the average person is conditioned to ignore the symptoms or consider these side effects as "normal."

These stressers are toxic and load the liver as well as the immune system. In order to boost the immune system and begin to build optimal health, these toxins must be cleansed and eliminated from the body.

The average person already uses all the energy available. As a result, the extra energy needed for this cleansing activity is not available. Consequently these toxins are not removed from the body and the body continues to accumulate toxic waste and eventually crashes under this toxic burden.

Excessive alcohol
Consumption of alcohol and beer not only impacts the immune system, it also increases fermentation levels in the gut. This is a disaster to anyone experiencing Candida. The internal fermentation produced by these beverages only adds to the Candida problem.

STRESSER 2 – NUTRITIONAL DEFICIENCIES
Green produce
Most produce today is not picked fresh from a backyard garden. Instead, it is picked green, shipped cross country (sometimes even

from other countries) and stacked onto shelves at a grocery store. When produce is picked green, the phytochemicals and essential saccharides are not allowed to fully develop. These "plant chemicals" are known to help the body fight cancer and to help boost the immune system.

Poor soil
In the past, a farmer let the soil lay fallow between crops. Crops were rotated and few chemicals were added. Today in the name of progress we have bypassed these natural principles and now use chemicals to increase production. Today's non-organic farming methods produce harvests that are lacking many minerals.

Synthetic supplements
Two schools of thought exist on supplementation. One approach is to use fractionated, synthetic supplements in megadoses. The other approach (and the one I espouse) is to use whole foods so that nutrients are in synergistic forms and much smaller doses. The best source of research on this topic can be found in Judith deCava's book *The Real Truth About Vitamins and Minerals.*

STRESSER 3 – POOR DIGESTION AND ASSIMILATION
In order to digest and assimilate our food, we need to have an effective balance of digestive enzymes, pancreatic enzymes and hydrochloric acid. The increased use of antacids has lowered these digestive supports. The large consumption of fluids during mealtimes also hampers adequate digestion.

The most natural source of enzymes can be found in raw fruits and vegetables and/or juicing. A diet high in simple carbohydrates lacks enzymes and increases poor digestion.

STRESSER 4 – SLUGGISH LIVER
The liver is a major detox organ. With the increased toxic load coming from our environments, foods and lifestyles, the liver has become overburdened. This increased burden causes the liver to be sluggish which impacts its effective handling of toxins. The more

sluggish the liver becomes, the more the blood, digestive functions, immune functions and cleansing activities of the body are harmed.

STRESSER 5 – ADRENAL EXHAUSTION

Stress takes its toll on the body and the immune system. Stress can harm the immune system more than smoking, poor diet, lack of exercise and drug abuse. Stress lowers the effectiveness of every system in the body, especially the immune system.

When under stress, the body produces more of a hormone called adrenaline. When adrenaline is used to survive each day instead of infrequent emergencies, then the adrenals are positioned for exhaustion. Adrenal exhaustion goes beyond being tired. It moves into the realm of severe exhaustion or chronic fatigue.

STRESSER 6 – FUNGUS OVERGROWTH

Fungus overgrowth is the subject of this book. The existence of fungus overgrowth itself indicates a compromised immune system. The more overgrown the fungus becomes, the more the immune system is compromised. This sets a vicious cycle into operation. Once fungus is out of balance, then the bowel flora (good bacteria) is severely challenged and the body takes a major immune hit.

STRESSER 7 – FOOD SENSITIVITIES AND ALLERGIES

Food sensitivities are actually a response by the body to stress. Poor digestion and assimilation can trigger these sensitivities, as well as toxic burden and genetic predisposition. Specific antibodies get released with these reactions which impacts immune system functioning. Continuing to consume allergenic foods weakens the immune system, as well as stressing the hormone and digestive systems of the body.

STRESSER 8 – MINDSETS AND EMOTIONS

The spirit, soul and body are intimately related. Any optimal health program must take into consideration that God created us as a triune being. If a person believes in their heart that they are not worth being healthy, then they will consciously or unconsciously sabotage their best efforts to get healthy. Mindsets are reflected in belief systems and must be evaluated by both the individual and their health care provider.

Emotions play a big role in the health of the immune system. In my book, *Cleansing Made Simple,* I discuss the various organs and systems that are impacted by specific emotions. In addition to these emotions, the client's belief in any remedy and their belief in their health care provider will dramatically impact any results from a health protocol. According to your faith be it unto you!

STRESSER 9 – EXCESSIVE ANTIBIOTICS
Antibiotics destroy the good bacteria essential to the immune system, especially when the body is fighting Candidiasis. Today's use of antibiotics is excessive and unnecessary. Nowhere does that fact show more dramatically than in dealing with Candida. The very use of antibiotics, let alone their misuse, adds to the problem. Continued use almost nullifies the chance of removing Candida imbalances. The damage done by antibiotics is further discussed in the next chapter.

STRESSER 10 – LACK OF WATER
People consume more soda, coffee and tea than water. Yet, water is a key component of the body's fluids, the brain and body tissues. Water is necessary to keep our joints moving, our nutrients flowing, our body temperatures regulated and our waste byproducts eliminated. Approximately 50 to 60% of our total body weight consists of water. For the average person, that boils down to ten gallons.[4]

When a person asks me if tea or juice can replace their daily water intake, I respond with "*Water* is spelled differently than *tea* or *juice* because it is a different word and it *is* different! Water is water — pure and simple."

To determine how much water you need, first take your weight and divide it by two. This tells you how many ounces you should consume each day. For example if you weigh 150 pounds, you need to consume 75 ounces of water each day. To determine the number of glasses you need, take the 75 ounces and divide it by eight, which would be between nine and ten glasses of water each day.

In order to build the immune system, each of these stressers must be addressed. When you fail to recognize the existence and impact of these individual stressers, you lower your chance of success in destroying Candida. A healthy, well-functioning immune system is absolutely crucial in fighting and keeping Candida in balance!

Now that you have been given an overview of the ten most common stressers of the immune system, let's turn our attention to the immune system itself. Without at least a minimal working knowledge, you will sabotage the complex balancing of this intricate system.

People are not healed by herbs, supplements, medications or food. These supporters are merely tools in the hands of the immune system. Just as a hammer, set of nails and some lumber do not build a house, they are necessary for the builder to build the house.

Just as a contractor needs the right tools and raw materials to build a house, so your immune system requires the right tools to be well balanced and healthy. We want to support the immune system so that you can build your health and have the ability to successfully defeat Candida.

IMMUNE SYSTEM STRUCTURE

Your immune system is comprised of:

- ◆ organs and glands, such as the thymus, spleen and the bone marrow
- ◆ white blood cells, which include granulocytes, monocytes and lymphocytes (lymphocytes are broken into B cells, T cells and NK cells)
- ◆ the lymphatic system, which is comprised of vessels, fluid, nodes, the tonsils, adenoids and the appendix

- antibodies
- the complement system
- the skin

Without each of these members, the immune system is incomplete. Consequently any approach to build health must take each into consideration. The immune system is a marvelous orchestra that can play either beautiful music — as in health — or clang noisily — as in disease. You choose the music your immune system plays.

Only you can accept the responsibility for your health — whether it is poor or rich. When you divest yourself of that God-given responsibility of dominion over your body, you forfeit many rights and privileges. You join the ranks of many others who have come to accept poor health as "normal."

As you begin to study the immune system, it is not essential that you become an expert in your knowledge of each member. It is important, however, to begin to get a picture or understanding of how intricately interwoven the body is. Your body is not an isolated set of specialties. It is an intricate system that must be treated as a whole. Health remodeling must always be based on an appreciation of that fact.

Let's take a tour of your immune system and its various family members.

ORGANS AND GLANDS

Let's begin to learn about our wonderful immune systems by first looking at the various organs and glands that support immune system work.

Thymus — master gland

Located behind the breastbone, the thymus instructs the T cells (white blood cells that come from the thymus) what and when to attack. When the thymus is not efficient, harmful substances such as bacteria, viruses and cancer cells are not attacked and are left free to invade body tissues.

Sometimes thymus directions are so confused that some of the body's own cells attack the body itself. This is thought to be a consideration in arthritis and multiple sclerosis. Effective cell-to-cell communication is critical for effective thymus functioning.

In the past it was believed that the thymus became inactive after adolescence. Today, studies indicate that the thymus gland can be active past adolescence with proper diet, especially a diet rich in essential fatty acids. When the thymus is healthy past adolescence, the immune system can be further activated.

Spleen

The spleen produces, monitors, stores and destroys blood cells. It is a spongy, soft organ about the size of a hand formed into a fist. It is located in the upper part of the abdominal cavity, just under the rib cage on the left side. The white pulp is part of the immune system and the red pulp removes unwanted material from the blood. Lymphocytes (one type of white blood cells) can be produced and matured in the white pulp.

If the spleen is removed surgically, the body loses some of its ability to product protective antibodies and to remove unwanted bacteria from the blood. This in turn lowers the body's ability to fight infection. This function is then taken over by the liver. If the liver is already overloaded, this can tremendously impair the immune function.

Bone Marrow

Red blood cells, white blood cells and platelets are produced in the bone marrow. Within bone marrow, all blood cells originate from a single cell called a stem cell. When a stem cell divides, it first becomes a red blood cell, white blood cell or platelet-producing cell. These immature cells further divide and become mature white blood cells, red blood cells or platelets. The speed of production is based on the body's need. The bone marrow produces more white blood cells in response to levels of infections.

These organs and glands (thymus, spleen and bone marrow) are the boot camp for your immune system. Boot camp is designed to train, produce and equip military members to protect a country. These organs and glands train, produce and equip your cells, fluids and antibodies when and how to do their jobs.

When boot camp is sloppy, the soldiers are sloppy. When the effectiveness of these organs and glands are compromised, your cells, fluids and antibodies are greatly impacted and consequently your overall immune system is impacted.

WHITE BLOOD CELLS

White blood cells are not as numerous as red blood cells, but they are an integral part of your immune system. There is approximately one white cell for every 660 red blood cells. It is interesting to note that refined sugar has been shown to inhibit white blood cell immune functions in sensitive individuals.

White blood cells are like your knights in white armor. You don't need as many of them as the rest of the foot soldiers, but their presence is crucial to win any battle.

There are five types of white blood cells — granulocytes, monocytes, eosinophils, basophils and lymphocytes. Each type of white blood cell plays a key role in immune functioning. Let's take a look at each of these types of white blood cells so that you can appreciate the type of army these cells provide.

Granulocytes

Also called neutrophils, granulocytes are the most prevalent of the white blood cells. They help protect the body against bacterial and fungal infections and ingest foreign debris. These cells are like packmen ... they eat and they attack. Their specialty includes bacteria and fungus.

Monocytes

Monocytes ingest dead or damaged cells and provide immunologic defenses against many infective organisms. Another type of packmen, monocytes both eat and defend against infection. When invaders have had time to multiply and infect, monocytes help eat away at the enemy.

Eosinophils

Eosinophils kill parasites, destroy cancer cells and are involved in allergenic responses. Since parasites are often associated with Candida, it is important to have eosinophils killing these unhealthy "critters." In addition, it is the eosinophils that recognize and kill cancer cells and help the body handle allergenic responses.

Basophils

Basophils are fewer in number but they play a key role in helping the body handle allergic responses.

Lymphocytes

Even though lymphocytes are relatively small in size, they are the main cells of the lymphatic system. Lymphocytes can live for years or even decades. These are the warriors that fight the war on disease day in and day out. These cells carry much valuable information, if their computer banks are not tampered with by internal computer bugs.

Lymphokines are the chemical messengers (hormones) produced by lymphocytes to strengthen and regulate a series of defensive and offensive immune actions. These messengers carry the secret code to war on how to defeat any invasion.

Lymphocytes are composed of T cells, B cells and NK (Natural Killer) cells. T and B cells circulate throughout the bloodstream and lymphatic vessels. They can also be found in the spleen, lymph nodes, tonsils, intestines and mucus-secreting surfaces. They can also be found in connective tissues throughout the body.

The Lymphocytes are like the Navy, they navigate through body fluids to kill the enemy. They take some R and R in various islands (the spleen, nodes, tonsils, etc.) to clean up and restore themselves. They can go anywhere and they are crucial in the overall war on disease.

T cells

T cells make and secrete cytokines (chemical messengers) after binding to other cells. They then give orders to the rest of the immune system as to how to fight that particular infection. T cells originate in the thymus of a fetus, hence the name *T* cells. T cells interpret information and communicate with all other lymphocytes through numerous chemical responses.

T cells are long-lived. With adequate nutrient support they become memory cells so that whenever they spot a future exposure to the same agent, they initiate an even faster and more vigorous immune response.

Without strong T cells your immune system's memory is greatly compromised. When the T cells are weak or confused, they can give wrong directions and actually cause the body to go to war against itself. This results in internal cannibalism ... the body destroys itself from within!

B cells

B cells protect the body by both producing antibodies that fight infections directly and by aiding other cells to kill microorganisms. B cells require signals from T helper cells to produce optimal antibodies. B cells originate in bone marrow, hence the name *B* cells.

You want your B cells to be healthy, not enablers or sabotagers. Their knowledge of antibodies is essential to how your immune system selects the right "recipe" to kill the enemy. The wrong recipe or instructions could feed the enemy instead of killing it.

NK cells

NK cells (natural killer cells) are slightly larger than T and B cells. All cell surface receptors are composed of glycoproteins which act as the language between the cells of the body (cell-to-cell communication). The glycoproteins on the cell membrane can be thought of as individual letters and words. *Glyco* is Greek for sugar and proteins are the combination of amino acids. Glycoproteins are cell surface molecules composed of proteins and sugars. Without adequate glyconutrients ("sugar nutrients") NK cells dysfunction and the correct chemical messengers are not released through the immune system.

They originate in the bone marrow and ultimately represent 5 to 10% of the total lymphocytes cells in the blood. NK cells are made up of glycoproteins and are prone to dysfunction when deficient in glyconutrients. NK cells secrete several chemical messengers and immune system hormones.

These messengers communicate with the entire immune system, helping to regulate the activities of the entire system. A complex system of multiple messages works throughout the immune system. The NK cells act as important intermediary signaling cells for this messaging process.

NK cells are totally dependent on good cell-to-cell communication. They are released to kill upon conception. Without accurate directions these killers are as dangerous to the body as a field of mines. NK cells go where the action is and their main mission is to kill. Only good cell-to-cell communication ensures they kill the right enemy.

THE LYMPHATIC SYSTEM

The lymphatic system is separate from our arteries and veins, but anatomically adjacent and intimately related. It serves as a transport system for nutrients absorbed from the gastrointestinal tract (GI tract). The lymph takes these nutrients to the cells. If the nutrients cannot pass through the GI tract, then the cells are not nourished. Likewise, if foreign objects pass through the GI tract, they too go to the cells throughout the body.

The lymph also works as a drainage system for foreign organisms and matter that have escaped the bloodstream or are too large to enter it. Once these foreign organisms are trapped in lymph nodes, they are attacked and eliminated by immune cells. The lymph vessels take the toxic waste from the tissues and cells, through the nodes and dump it out of the body via the skin, bowel and kidneys.

The lymphatic system is composed of the fluid which is carried by the vessels, the nodes, the tonsils/adenoids and the appendix. This fluid is not pumped through the vessels as the blood is pumped through the body. Instead, the lymphatic system must be stimulated through exercise (especially rebounders or mini trampolines), deep breathing, massage and skin brushing.

Of all the body's systems, the lymphatic system is most impacted by suppressed emotions. When the lymphatic system is out of balance, it can manifest as excess mucus (i.e., sinus issues, ear aches, asthma, etc.), stopped drainage (i.e., post nasal drip, puffiness, etc.) or impaired lymph vessel integrity.

Since the lymphatic system is virtually half of the immune system, these imbalances impact overall immune function. With any health protocol, it is essential that the lymph be opened so that nutrition and toxins can be effectively transported. In addition to the needed nutrition and supplementation, it is also important to look at any suppressed emotions that could be aggravating the situation.

Lymphatic fluid
Lymphatic fluid (rich in white blood cells) flows through the lymphatic vessels. It returns water, proteins, toxins and other substances from the body's tissues to the blood stream. All substances absorbed by the lymph pass through at least one lymph node and its filtering mesh of lymphocytes. Over half of our total lymphatic fluid is produced by hepatocytes (liver cells).

Lymph nodes
Lymph nodes contain a mesh of tissue in which lymphocytes are tightly packed. This mesh of lymphocytes filters, attacks and destroys harmful organisms that cause infections. Lymph nodes are often clustered in areas where the lymphatic vessels branch off, such as the neck, armpits and groin. Other locations include the areas around the knees, liver, spleen and intestines.

The term *swollen glands* is a term commonly used to describe enlargement of the lymph nodes or glands of the neck. Technically it can refer to the enlargement of any node (i.e., nodes in armpit or groin). The enlargement of a node is a signal of an infection in that area since the job of the nodes is to filter out microscopic material to help prevent the spread of infection.

If a person does a cleanse and experiences healing crisis symptoms (i.e., aching in the limbs, nausea, headaches, etc.), then almost always it is an indication of an overburden in the nodes. If the nodes swell, either in the neck, armpits or groin area, this further underscores the fact that the body is especially toxic. It is crucial that some type of lymphatic support be added to the cleanse program as well as slowing the actual cleanse. At this point it is not better to keep pushing. Detoxing too fast can create as many problems as the toxic load itself.

In my research and practice, I have found that people who are missing tonsils and appendix (lymph nodes) require longer periods of time to rebuild lymphatic system health.

Appendix

The appendix is a small, finger-shaped tube projecting from the large intestine near the point where it joins the small intestine. Part of the lymphatic system, it serves as a mesh of lymphocytes which filter, attack and destroy harmful organisms that cause infections. When it is over burdened, the infection can erupt into appendicitis.

A simple way to view the appendix is to view it as an air traffic controller. It directs the flow of toxins found in the body below the waist. Without the appendix, the lymphatic system must improvise in some of its directions. Obviously we don't want a sick controller functioning in the body. However, it does serve a purpose and to remove it without a good reason is foolish.

Tonsils/Adenoids

The tonsils are located at the back of the mouth and the adenoids at the back of the nasal cavity. Tonsils and adenoids consist of lymph tissues and help fight off infections.

The tonsils serve as another set of air traffic controllers. They direct the flow of toxins found in the body above the waist. People who have had their tonsils removed often have problems with their shoulders and necks and tend to be more vulnerable to infections. I had my tonsils removed at age five and have experienced problems with my shoulders and neck for years. I worked on my lymphatic system for well over twelve months before I was able to see significant progress.

Infected tonsils (or adenoids or appendix) are simply an indication of the toxic load the lymphatic system is attempting to handle. Instead of just removing these nodes, a health conscious person should realize the body is in desperate need of cleansing. The cleansing manner selected must be in a safe manner that is paced to the body's ability to handle the toxic load.

If you are missing your tonsils, adenoids and/or appendix, be sure to work with a qualified health care provider to begin supporting your lymphatic system. The lymph support measures discussed later in this book are an ideal place to start. Don't assume you have no problem — your lymphatic system does need support. Don't wait for the crisis to begin to provide that support.

ANTIBODIES
Antibodies are matured B cells that are stimulated by antigens (any substance that causes the body to produce an antibody). Once again cell-to-cell communication is crucial for this process. If the body is unable to recognize a foreign substance, no antibody will be produced. If cell-to-cell communication is off, the wrong antibody can be produced or produced in an incorrrect manner. The result of any of these failures is a reduced immune reaction when it is needed.

Antibodies, along with other molecules (i.e., complement, interferons, interleukins and cytokines), are required to keep Candida in check through binding and/or killing procedures.

In order for antibodies and these other molecules to function properly, a complex set of steps must be taken to produce the correct responses and sequences. Glyconutrients, comprised of a variety of saccharides (naturally occurring sugars) constitute a newly recognized nutrient group used by the body for cellular synthesis.[5]

Antibodies are also known as immunoglobins (Ig) and are the primarily cellular secretions of the immune system. Immunoglobins are broken into four primary categories: IgA, IgG, IgM and IgE.

When there is low antibody production (which often will not show until ages 10 to 20), then various autoimmune disorders can begin to show. These disorders include adrenal failure (Addison's disease), thyroiditis and rheumatic arthritis.

It is possible to have a deficiency in any one class of antibodies instead of all the antibodies. The most common deficiency is in IgA, which can cause chronic respiratory infections and allergies.

IgA

IgA is the antibody that plays an important role in the body's defenses against the invasion of microorganisms through mucous membrane-lined surfaces. IgA is found in secretions such as milk, saliva, tears, respiratory and intestinal secretions. It works to contain localized infection from spreading throughout the body.

IgG

IgG is the most prevalent type of antibody and is present in both the blood and the tissues. It is the only antibody that is transferred across the placenta from mother to fetus. The mother's IgG protects the fetus and newborn until the infant's immune system can produce its own antibodies.

IgM

IgM is the antibody that is produced upon exposure to an antigen such as vaccinations. IgM is abundant in the blood but not normally found in organs or tissues.

IgE

IgE is the antibody that causes immediate allergic reactions such as hay fever, asthma and hives. It can cause more harm than good. It can be helpful in fighting against parasitic infections.

THE COMPLEMENT SYSTEM

The body's Complement System is composed of eighteen plasma proteins which are vital to the body's defense. This important system consists of two parts. Part one is the classical, which battles autoimmune disease. Part two is the alternative pathway which fights infection.

The Skin

The skin serves as a primary barrier to infection along with the linings of the mouth, the gastrointestinal tract, respiratory tract (nostrils, sinuses, bronchioles and lungs) and the genitourinary tract. In a state of well being, these rapidly reproducing cells of our skin and tract linings prevent attachment and penetration by infectious agents. The mucus is a protective agent that lines the cells.

Summary

If the immune system is stressed, infections and disease may take over. Often people wait to have a disease before they realize they have a problem. The following symptoms are indicators of chronic infection and should signal the need to build the immune system.

- pale, thin appearance
- skin rash
- pustules (pus filled pimples)
- eczema
- broken blood vessels
- hair loss
- purple blotches
- redness of the lining of the eye
- enlarged lymph nodes, such as those in the neck, armpits and groin
- scared and perforated eardrums
- crusted nostrils from discharge
- enlarged liver and spleen
- redness around the anus from chronic diarrhea

If you or your children show these symptoms, even if you currently have no signs of a disease, then your immune system is already compromised. The more compromised it becomes the higher the guarantee that you will deal with a health crisis. The only question remaining is which type of health crisis you will experience and when it will occur.

Don't wait for the crisis! Learn how to boost the immune system, even if you aren't facing the crisis or a Candida episode!

NOTES FOR CHAPTER ONE

1. Darryl See, Ph.D., *Breakthrough Discoveries in Immune System Disorders* (Visua.Com: 1998), p. 14.

2. Michael T. Murray, N.D. and Jade Beutler, R.R.T., R.C.T., *Understanding Fats & Oils* (Encinatas, CA: Progressive Health Publishing, 1996), pp. 1 – 2.

3. Ann Louise Gittleman, M.S., C.N.S., *Get the Sugar Out* (New York: Crown Trade Paperbacks, 1996), p. xiii.

4. Gordon S. Tessler, Ph.D., *Breaking the Fat Barrier* (Raleigh, NC: Be Well Publications, 1993), p. 43.

5. *Special Report: Effect of Aloe Polymannose and Glyconutritionals on Candida*, Proceedings of the Fisher Institute for Medical Research: February, 1999, vol. 1, no. 1.

REFERENCES FOR CHAPTER ONE

SM Fu and HG Kunkel, "Membrane Immunoglovulin of B Lymphocytes," *J Exp Med*: 1974, 140:894 – 903.

GP Ross, MJ Polley and EM Rabellino, "Two Different Complement Receptors on Human Lymphocytes," *J Exp Med*: 1973, 138:798 – 818.

WJ Storkus and JR Dawson, "Target Structures Involved in Natural Killing (NK): Characteristics, Distribution and Candidate Molecules," *Critical Reviews in Immunology*: 1990, 10:393 – 416.

Two
Candida Defined
♦♦♦

Candida albicans is a type of parasitic yeast-like fungus that inhabits the intestines, genital tract, mouth, esophagus and throat. Normally this fungus lives in balance with other bacteria and yeasts in the body. In a healthy person a large portion of the good bacteria includes lactobacilli, which are friendly bacteria that help fight unfriendly bacteria, high cholesterol levels and even some cancers.

Unlike these good bacteria, the Candida albicans are usually only present in small numbers. They are single cell funguses that belong to the vegetable kingdom. They are cousins of the molds that live in damp basements, wood stumps and old buildings.

In a healthy, balanced body, Candida albicans are harmless. However, when certain conditions exist (excessive stress or lowered immune function), then this delicate balance is broken and an imbalance known as Candidiasis occurs. When imbalance strikes the out-of-control yeast-like fungus travels through the bloodstream to many parts of the body. It is estimated that Candida affects one out of three Americans.

Many other factors can contribute to and/or cause a manifestation of Candida. The factors we will quickly review include:

♦ food allergies
♦ antibiotic usage

- birth control pill usage
- children (thrush, diaper rash, ear infections and swollen tonsils)
- infertility
- chronic fatigue syndrome
- parasites
- blood types
- amalgam fillings

CANDIDA AND FOOD ALLERGIES

Candidiasis can lead to many problems, including severe gastrointestinal disorders which can lead to malabsorption and malnutrition. Candidiasis is often undiagnosed in the medical community since it can mimic food allergies and other food-related maladies. Unlike food allergies, which are often due to a lack of hydrochloric acid or digestive enzymes, the fungus of Candidiasis permits the allergic substances to penetrate the blood steam. This promotes food-allergy reactions that enzymes or hydrochloric acid will not effectively address.

An allergy or sensitivity is an inappropriate response by the body's immune system to a substance that is not normally harmful. Once again, it is a balanced immune system that keeps allergies and sensitivities in check. When the communication system of the immune system is out of balance, it is possible for the body to react to "normal" foods, substances and chemicals with uncomfortable symptoms.

The substances that cause these symptoms are called allergens. Although any substance can cause a reaction, some allergens are more common than others. They include:

- pollen
- dust
- cosmetics
- animal hair and dander
- insect venom

- some prescription drugs
- molds

The most common food allergens include:

- chocolate
- dairy
- wheat
- eggs
- shellfish
- strawberries
- corn
- soy

Food allergies and food intolerances are not the same. An intolerance is usually based on a deficiency in digestion which is usually due to a lack of enzymes. A food allergy occurs when a person's immune system generates an antibody response to an ingestion of a certain food(s). Food intolerances can eventually lead to food allergies.

Reactions to food allergies can be immediate or delayed. The more delayed the reaction, the more difficult it can be to trace. Allergies do tend to run in families. It is believed that children who are not breastfed are often more likely to develop allergies.

FOOD ALLERGY PULSE TEST
If you suspect that you are sensitive or allergic to a specific food, the following test can be taken.

1. Sit in a comfortable chair and relax. Take your resting pulse by counting the number of beats in a sixty-second period. (Or take the rate in ten seconds and multiply by six.) A normal pulse rate is 52 to 70 beats per minute.
2. Consume the suspected food in its purest form (i.e., test cream of wheat instead of bread which contains wheat, yeast and a sweetener).

---

3. Wait 15 to 20 minutes.
4. Take your pulse again. If your pulse rate has increased more than ten beats per minute, omit this food from your diet for one month.

The Candida diet removes many of the common allergens (i.e., wheat, dairy, etc.). If you find that you have stomach pains during the Candida diet, it is possible that additional allergenic foods are being consumed that need to be eliminated. The least expensive method of identifying allergens is to keep a food diary (tracking actual food intake along with emotional, mental and physical symptoms) or taking the allergy pulse. Blood tests and/or working with an allergist can also be of help.

During the Candida cleanse, it is highly recommended that you remove any offending foods and add the appropriate digestive support (i.e., digestive enzymes, vegetable juicing, probiotics and/or hydrochloric acid support).

CANDIDA AND ANTIBIOTICS

Candida overgrowth often comes as a result of excessive use of antibiotics. This excess is a contributor whether that excess comes from personal antibiotic prescriptions or from eating animal-based products from animals that have been given antibiotics. Antibiotics, whether they are taken directly for medical reasons or ingested indirectly through antibiotic-fed livestock or the water supply, kill the beneficial intestinal microflora bacteria that normally control Candida.[1]

Are antibiotics really over-prescribed? Research shows that gynecologists prescribe 2,645,000 antibiotics per week. Over $500 million per year is spent on antibiotics for ear infections. Congressional hearings have shown that 40% to 60% of all antibiotic prescriptions are misprescribed.[2]

Joseph Pizzorno, N.D. in his book *Total Wellness* says that "When patients receive antibiotics, the level of Candida in their intestines increases so much and the intestines become so damaged, that pieces of the Candida leak into their blood and inhibit the function of their immune system."[3]

At one time it was believed that persistent and recurrent infections were responsive to antibiotics. However, it is now believed that the increased and excessive use of antibiotics causes resistance to antibiotics and an increasing incidence of yeast infections especially from the Candida albicans.[4]

The entire process of getting infections (the initial reason for taking antibiotics) is due to a compromised immune system. There is an alternative to covering up the symptoms of infection and/or killing off bacteria (the bad and the good) through the use of antibiotics. Building the immune system can reduce the need for antibiotics and consequently their negative effects. A strong immune system helps prevent occurrences of bacteria and keeps the Candida albicans in balance.

CANDIDA AND BIRTH CONTROL PILLS

Birth control pills change the vaginal flora and can increase the likelihood of yeast infections and Candida. When birth control pills are being taken, or have been taken, along with antibiotics, it is quite common for a woman to have Candida.

Prior to the pill, one out of four cases of vaginitis was due to the Candida fungus. Today, nine out of ten cases of vaginitis are Candida related and there are many more cases of this condition since the advent of the Pill.

The most common reason for putting women on birth control pills is not for birth control, it is to help regulate menstrual cycles. Unbalanced hormones often accompany Candida problems. Bringing the Candida under control while boosting the body's natural hormonal cycle (I highly recommend our *Raging Hormones* audio tape series) can help resolve this problem without the use of birth control pills.

If the reason for taking birth control pills is to actually prevent pregnancy, then other methods should be considered. In 1995 the National Survey of Family Growth showed that only 3% of all contraception users chose natural birth control. The top three methods used were: sterilization (27.7%), the pill (26.9%) and condoms (20.4%). Few doctors promote any natural options.

Natural birth control method goes beyond the old-fashioned rhythm method. Can this method work? It does take more knowledge and time, but it also has fewer consequences. A New Zealand study published in the *Journal of Advances in Contraception* (June 1997) found that 90% of users were highly satisfied with natural birth control, citing effectiveness, a heightened awareness of their overall health and freedom from drugs as major benefits. For more information on natural birth control, check out the resources listed in Appendix E.

CANDIDA AND CHILDREN

Children are prone to Candida as their immune systems are immature. Antibiotics are often given to infants, sometimes inappropriately, which increases the chances of Candida. In addition, babies frequently pick up Candida when they pass through the birth canal if the mom has Candida.

A breast-fed baby is known to have higher levels of antibodies and a higher immune system. Research shows that five of the eight essential saccharides (glyconutrients) exist in breast milk. These five saccharides are produced by enzymatic attachments of residues to lactose (milk sugar). Research has shown that breast-fed babies have fewer incidents of eczema (symptoms of Candida), asthma (excess mucous), diarrhea and ear infections.

The average American does not regularly get six or seven of these in his diet. The two sugars that are normally consumed include glucose and galactose. These two sugars can be converted into the other essential sugars, but the process is based on a large number of enzymatic steps. Due to stress and toxicity, the enzymatic process often breaks down, leaving the body short of these essential glyconutrients.

An alternative to having a deficiency of these essential sugars (critical to cell membrane function) is to breast feed babies and include glyconutrient support in a daily supplement protocol (see Appendix A for recommendations). For more information on glyconutrient support, check out the website of Dr. Daryl See, one of the leading immunologists at electriciti.com/edison/drsee.

In addition to the essential saccharides, breast milk also has a high content of natural antibodies that encourage the growth of lactobacilli in the infant's digestive system. Breast-fed babies have a significantly lower incidence of respiratory tract infections, ear infections, systemic Candida and Candida of the mouth (thrush).[5]

THRUSH

Yeast infections can also cause thrush. Thrush appears as white, flaky, cheesy-looking patches covering all or part of the tongue and gums, the inside of the cheeks and, sometimes, the lips. These patches do not scrape off easily. When scraped off, they may leave a red, inflamed area that can bleed. Thrush can often cause a child to lose her appetite.

A child with thrush, can cause the nursing mother to get the thrush on her nipples. Nipples with a thrush infection will be red, swollen, tender and possibly cracked. They may also itch, flake and/or burn.

DIAPER RASH

Diaper rash can be caused by many things. If it is due to Candida, the skin will be smooth, shiny and bright red. The borders of the lesions and rash will be well defined and there may be scattered spots in the groin area.

EAR INFECTION

Ear infections are among the most common infections in toddlers. In fact, Dr. Balch in his book *Prescription for Nutritional Healing* says that as many as 95% of all children have at least one ear infection by the age of six. The most common prescription for an ear infection is an antibiotic.

There are several different types of ear infections. External otitis (outer ear infection) is an acute infection that is often preceded by an upper respiratory infection or allergies. The ear canal becomes inflamed and swollen. Symptoms can include fever, ear discharge, pain and throbbing.

Middle ear (otitis media) infections are very common in children and infants. This infection resides behind the eardrum where the small bones of the ear are located. Symptoms include earache; sharp, dull or throbbing pains; pressure in the ear and high fever. High altitudes and cold temperatures can increase discomfort.

Frequent middle ear infections affect 30% or more of children under the age of six. A common cause of these ear infections is allergies. I have also found an excess of mucus (often associated with the food allergens of wheat and dairy) also contributes to the infections.

Working with the Candida diet, boosting the immune system and using aged garlic can be an effective alternative to the constant use of antibiotics. Excellent resources are available to help parents address this problem naturally. Please see Appendix D for recommended reading materials.

SWOLLEN TONSILS

Swollen tonsils often exist when there is excess mucus in the middle ear. The swollen tonsils can obstruct the Eustachian tube, thereby preventing the middle ear from draining properly. Some doctors believe that removing the tonsils will resolve this problem.

The tonsils are essential lymphoid structures that play a key role in protecting the ear, nose and throat areas from bacteria, fungi and viruses. Removing the tonsils may increase the child's vulnerability to microorganisms, especially yeast.

A more natural alternative to removing tonsils is to build the immune system (see Appendix A) , help the glands drain (via the use of lymph drainage homeopathics — see Appendix A) and follow the Candida diet.

I have worked with many parents who chose this approach. These parents were pleased to note that not only did the swelling subside, but many other "normal" complaints subsided. Those complaints included colds, tummy aches and hyperactivity. I can attest to many of these changes since I watched a child transform from the child terror our office wanted outlawed to a nice child the office enjoyed.

CANDIDA AND INFERTILITY

Infertility is a rising problem. It is now estimated that infertility affects 20% of all American couples. As women are under more and more stress, experience higher toxic and increased hormonal imbalances, their ability to get pregnant seems to drop. It is almost as if the body is saying that it does not have the energy reserves to handle the high cost of nourishing two bodies — Mom and baby. These factors — stress, toxic load and hormonal imbalances — also play a role in Candida.

Sidney MacDonald Baker, M.D. in his book *Detoxification & Healing: The Key to Optimal Health* says "The endocrine effects of Candida are dramatic, and infertility, in my experience, is a common consequence."[6]

Many times women who change their lifestyle habits through eating a more balanced diet, exercising and reducing stress will find themselves pregnant. A common factor to infertility seems to be a high intake of sugar, which of course feeds Candida. Medical testing evaluates many factors, but the high intake of sugar is almost always overlooked.

Cleansing the body and changing the diet are far less expensive in both money and energy than many of the high-tech intervention methods. The cleansing and diet changes can help men with low sperm count as much as it can be of help to the women.

CANDIDA AND CFS

In 1989 and 1990, Carol Jessop, M.D., a California researcher of CFS (Chronic Fatigue Syndrome) and Assistant Clinical Professor at the University of California at San Francisco, presented case studies of patients with chronic fatigue syndrome. She reported that 80% had histories of recurrent antibiotic treatment.

William G. Crook, M.D., author of *Chronic Fatigue Syndrome and the Yeast Connection*, concludes similarly that overuse of antibiotics is a major contributing factor to the development of chronic fatigue. Once again with the overuse of antibiotics, the presence of Candida can also accompany CFS.

Almost without exception research has shown that CFS affects more women than men. Women between the ages of 20 to 45 are most likely to develop the CFS disorder. The higher rate of Candida in women may explain the link for higher occurrences of CFS in women.[7]

So why do women experience this link between CFS and Candida more than men? The following facts explain this correlation.

+ Hormonal changes associated with normal menstrual cycles encourage yeast growth.
+ Birth control pills and pregnancy contribute to increased yeast growth.
+ Yeasts thrive in the warm, interior vaginal membranes.
+ Women tend to take more antibiotics as they notice health issues more frequently than men.

CFS has many symptoms including aching muscles and joints, anxiety, depression, difficulty concentrating, fever, headaches, intestinal problems, irritability, loss of appetite, mood swings, sleep disturbances, swollen glands and extreme fatigue. Symptoms often mimic those of flu or viral infections making it hard to diagnose.

It is found that CFS can reoccur if the root issues are not resolved. Candida cleansing and diet changes can be helpful in resolving CFS symptoms. Building the immune system is crucial in preventing reoccurrence of CFS. Chapter Six and Appendix A give you many options to build the immune system.

CANDIDA AND PARASITES

In 1976, the Center for Disease Control in Atlanta found one out of every six Americans had parasites. Other research indicates those numbers could be even higher. In a healthy person, the normal production of hydrochloric acid and pancreatic enzymes controls this problem. When a person is not healthy, has pets, travels internationally or eats food that has been prepared in an unclean manner, it is common to find parasites.

Parasites alter the immune system by neutralizing beneficial enzymes and releasing toxic enzymes which kill white blood cells. Consequently when parasites exist, a person is much more likely to have Candida.

A swollen belly (child or adult) often indicates the presence of parasites. If symptoms and/or testing indicate the presence of parasites, then a parasite cleanse should be included prior to or after a Candida cleanse (see Appendix A for parasite cleanse information).

CANDIDA AND BLOOD TYPES

Although some people find blood type analysis to be controversial when applied to foods, I have found it to be helpful. There are four basic blood types — Type O, Type A, Type B and Type AB. It is one of the antigens (see Chapter One) in the body that determines a person's blood type. A person's blood type is a crucial part of the immune system's security system.[8]

The chemical structure of blood types project out from the surface of the cells like antennae. These antennae are made from long chains of the sugars (glyconutrients). Type O contains the basic sugar fucose. Type A is formed when fucose combines with N-acetyl-galactosamine, another sugar. Type B is formed when fucose combines with D-galactosamine. Type AB is formed when fucose combines with the other two sugars N-acetyl-galactosamine and D-galactosamine.

Since these sugars are not found in an average diet, they must be made from the two common sugars glucose and galactose. Adding glyconutrient (essential sugar) support to the body helps support the blood and its antibody-building function.

Why is this support important? When your blood type antigen senses the presence of a foreigner, it creates an antibody. The plan of the antibody is to identify, tag and destroy the foreigner. This is why your blood type is important when you are considering surgery or blood transfusions. Mixing antigens will dangerously impact the immune system's ability to produce effective antibodies. The research of Dr. Karl Landsteiner, an Austrian physician and scientist of the early 1900's, identified blood types and their impact on transfusions.

The following review of each of the four blood types will give you a basic understanding of the foods that benefit overall health and those that should be avoided so as to not distract from overall health as it relates to Candida. Following these guidelines can be of help as you customize a Candida diet and plan an appropriate maintenance strategy.

In our metabolic profile planning done at Lifestyle for Health, we combine a person's blood type with his ancestry and a basic metabolic profile to determine a thoroughly balanced food plan. For more information on this type of food planning, I recommend Ann Louise Gittleman's book *Your Body Knows Best* and my *Meals in 30 Minutes.*

If you do not know your blood type and want to know it, you can find out by donating blood, checking with your physician or by contacting Dr. D'Adamo at North American Pharmacal, Inc. See Appendix E.

TYPE O BLOOD

Type O is the most common (85%) of all blood types in America. Persons with this blood type:

- ♦ Thrive on animal protein. (High intake of animal protein containing steroids and antibiotics increases the likelihood of Candida.)
- ♦ Have strong digestion, immune system and natural defenses against infections.
- ♦ Are sensitive to blood clotting, inflammatory diseases (i.e., arthritis), low thyroid, ulcers and allergies.
- ♦ Need vigorous exercise.

- Lose weight by:

Consuming less	Consuming more
wheat	kelp
corn	seafood
kidney beans	liver
navy beans	organic red meat
lentils, cabbage	kale
Brussels sprouts	spinach
cauliflower	broccoli
mustard greens	
dairy	

- Must balance protein consumption with appropriate vegetables to avoid over-acidification which can cause ulcers.
- Find walnuts and almonds beneficial, but not cashews, pistachios or peanuts.
- Do not do well with many of the Candida-restricted foods (including vinegar, pickled foods and corn syrup).
- May need additional vitamin B support, calcium, thyroid support (endocrine), DGL (de-glycyrrhizinated licorice to help reduce stomach acid) and pancreatic enzyme support.
- Develop more allergic-type hypersensitivity to Candida. It is especially important to restrict grains in Type Os who have yeast overgrowth.

TYPE A BLOOD

Persons with this blood type:

- Flourish on a vegetarian diet.
- Have sensitive digestive systems and are vulnerable to microbial ("critter") invasions.
- Do better on organic, fresh, pure, less-processed foods.
- Function the opposite of Type O; animal protein slows down the metabolism of a Type A. Meat is stored as fat due to his poor digestion and low stomach-acid content.
- Can have insulin imbalances due to consuming excessive amounts of wheat.

- Lose weight by:

Consuming less	Consuming more
meat	vegetable oils
dairy	soy foods
kidney beans	vegetables
Lima beans	pineapple
wheat	
processed meats	

- Fail to tolerate most dairy due to antibody composition of Type A, although goat products are sometimes tolerated.
- Tend to produce more mucus which feeds Candida.
- Should avoid vinegar, which feeds Candida.
- Need additional immune building support, stress-reducing support (endocrine system support), probiotics (good bacteria) and antioxidant support in a supplement plan.
- Have a tough time eradicating yeast overgrowth, especially after antibiotic use.

TYPE B BLOOD

Persons with this blood type:

- Are more like Type O than Type A.
- Tend toward diabetes, CFS and autoimmune diseases, such as Lou Gehrig's disease, MS and lupus.
- More commonly have hypoglycemia, yet "grazing" does not work as well for this blood type.
- Lose weight by:

Consuming less	Consuming more
corn	green vegetables
lentils	meat
peanuts	eggs
sesame seeds	liver
buckwheat	
wheat	

- Do better on red meat, turkey, pheasant, lamb but not chicken.

- Tend to do well on dairy products, due to the presence of the milk sugar (D-galactosamine) except for some ethnic backgrounds (i.e., African American).
- Need to watch tomato-based food (as well as corn) — these can irritate Type B's stomach linings.
- Can have Candida triggered by mold-containing foods, such as olives.
- Need additional immune support, magnesium, phytochemicals, digestive enzymes and mental clarity support (i.e., flaxseed oil, ginkgo biloba) and lecithin.
- Are the least likely to get Candida of all four blood types. When Candida does exist, it is essential to omit wheat.
- Although only 9% of all Americans are Type B, 30% to 40% of all self-made millionaires are Type B! Chinese and Jewish populations tend to be Type B.

TYPE AB BLOOD

Type AB is the most rare blood type. Persons with this blood type:

- Have sensitive digestive tracts and tend toward microbial ("critter") invasions.
- Have health risks which include cancer, heart disease and anemia.
- Lose weight by:

Consuming less	*Consuming more*
red meat	tofu
kidney beans	seafood
Lima beans	dairy
seeds	green vegetables
corn	kelp
buckwheat	pineapple
wheat	

- Need animal protein, although beef and chicken should be avoided and animal protein portions should be small.
- Usually digest dairy, especially yogurt and eggs, well.
- Should consume seeds in small amounts and with caution.

- ♦ Should avoid wheat if mucus conditions such as asthma or frequent infections exist.
- ♦ Do better with rice than pasta.
- ♦ Seem to do better with tomatoes than any other blood type.
- ♦ Need additional immune building support, antioxidants (phytochemicals, Vitamin C and zinc) and a digestive enzyme with dairy support.
- ♦ Have a tough time eradicating yeast overgrowth, especially after antibiotic use. Improved glyconutrient support is important to boost the immune function.

Following the Candida diet with the appropriate blood type considerations will not only help ensure overall success, but also a better approach for weight balancing. Utilizing the nutrient support suggestion is helpful in identifying a maintenance plan after completing the Candida cleanse.

CANDIDA AND AMALGAM FILLINGS

The hazards of silver-mercury fillings have been discussed, criticized, mocked and challenged over the years. The American Dental Association, which represents approximately 75% of the nation's dentists, continues to support the use of silver amalgams as safe.

However, there is a separate view that finds amalgams can be toxic and harmful. Alfred Zamm, M.D., of Kingston, New York wrote an article entitled "Anticandida Albicans Therapy: Is There Ever an End To It?, Dental Mercury Removal: An Effective Adjunct." In a conversation with Dr. Crook, Zamm said:

> Mercury from dental amalgam induces symptoms in a sensitive group of the population that has been observed to be sensitive to xenobiotic substances. This sensitive group serves as a marker of the potential danger of dental mercury to the rest of the population who are also at risk but may not yet exhibit symptoms. I've found that in many severely

ill patients, including those with chronic fatigue, Candidiasis and allergies that removal of silver/ mercury dental fillings is an effective way of improving their health.[9]

Since removing amalgams can be hard on the immune system, it is important to work with a biological dentist. This type of dentist understands that what is in the mouth impacts the entire body. He will also evaluate overall immune system strength, compatibility of composites and the sequence with which to remove fillings.

Several tests can be done to determine if mercury toxicity is a problem. One of the most common and least expensive is a hair or hair and nail analysis. These tests are often provided by nutritionists, chiropractors and other health care providers. Nails must be free of polish and hair must not have been chemically treated.

For more information on amalgams, contact the DAMS (Dental Amalgam Mercury Syndrome) non-profit organization at:

The International DAMS Newsletter
6025 Osuna Blvd., Suite B
Albuquerque, NM 87109
505-888-0111
Fax: 505-888-4554

CANDIDA AND EMOTIONS

One of the clients I worked with was making excellent progress by strictly following the Candida diet and the Candida cleanse. In the second month of her program she broke out with a severe vaginal infection. She checked with her doctor who did a biopsy and found nothing.

As I was talking with her, I felt led to ask if she had ever been sexually abused. She had been abused as a child and in marriage. Interestingly, the sexual abuse had surfaced during a counseling session only days before the infection occurred. Coincidence? I don't think so.

Sexual abuse is one of the questions our Stress Questionnaire asks. Frequently I see that box marked on the people who show other Candida symptoms. It took this client's situation for me to begin to see a possible relationship.

If a person has unresolved issues with past and/or current sexual abuse, they will often sabotage their efforts to successfully complete a Candida cleanse. Abuse often links to shame in a person's identity. At that point they do not believe they have value as a person and will not "allow" themselves to get healthy.

I am sure that there are many other emotions that impact the successful resolution of Candida. If a person continues to experience Candida after closely following the diet, the cleanse and appropriate supplementation, I suggest they look at emotional roots.

In my book *Discovering Wholeness,* I discuss the role of emotions and overall health. The two most devastating emotions appear to be fear and anger. Research shows that unresolved fear can manifest as asthma, respiratory problems, upper chest tightness, kidney problems and issues with women. Unresolved anger can settle in the liver, heart and impact issues with men.

Other unresolved emotions that have been linked to health problems include:

◆ bitterness	⇨	gall bladder
◆ guilt	⇨	shoulder problems
◆ control or hatred	⇨	colon
◆ loneliness	⇨	aches
◆ suppression	⇨	allergies
◆ hostility or unforgiveness	⇨	arthritis
◆ inadequate finances	⇨	lower back pain
◆ resentment	⇨	Candida
◆ despair	⇨	CFS
◆ nervousness	⇨	coughs
◆ need for protection	⇨	weight
◆ stress	⇨	headaches
◆ grief	⇨	lupus
◆ inflexibility	⇨	MS

- ♦ irritation   ⇨   skin problems
- ♦ insecurity   ⇨   stomach problems

The list could go on and on. It is important to realize that the associated emotion is not the source of the health issue, but it may be a contributor. A qualified counselor, prayer partner or friend may be of help to you in identifying, releasing and eliminating the emotional link to Candida or its many aliases.

NOTES FOR CHAPTER TWO

1. Michael A. Schmidt, Lendon H. Smith and Keith W. Sehnert, *Beyond Antibiotics* (Berkeley, CA: North Atlantic Books, 1994), pp. 55 – 57.

2. "Antibiotics Use Must Slow, Experts Warn," quote by Gail Cassell, VP of Eli Lilly & Co., *The Denver Post*: August 12, 1998.

3. Joseph Pizzorno, N.D., *Total Wellness* (Rocklin, CA: Prima Publishing, 1998), pp. 52 – 54.

4. Sidney MacDonald Baker, M.D., *Detoxification & Healing: The Key to Optimal Health* (New Canaan, CT: Keats Publishing, Inc., 1997), p. 156.

5. Mike Samuels, M.D. and Nancy Samuels, *The Well Baby Book* (New York: Simon & Schuster, 1991), p. 168.

6. *Detoxification & Healing: The Key to Optimal Health*, p. 156.

7. William G. Crook, M.D., *Chronic Fatigue Syndrome and the Yeast Connection* (Jackson, TN: Professional Books, 1992), p. 26.

8. J. D'Adamo, N.D., *Eat Right for Your Blood Type* (New York: G.P. Putnam's Sons, 1996), p. 18.

9. *Chronic Fatigue Syndrome and the Yeast Connection*, p. 333.

THREE
CANDIDA SYMPTOMS
✦✦✦

How do you know if you have Candida? Many symptoms can point to its existence. The more symptoms you have, the more likely that you have Candida. Most commonly associated symptoms of Candida are detailed below. I've also included a history and weighted symptom list to help you determine the likelihood of you having Candida.

Before we examine this list, let's answer some commonly asked questions.

1. Can a person take a medical test to determine the presence of Candida?
Yes. It is, however, possible to have Candida and not have it show in medical testing. The most common medical treatment for Candida includes anti-fungal medications, such as nystatin, ketoconazole and amphotericin. Unfortunately, the use of these meds on a repeated basis can lead to stronger strains of yeast that become drug resistant.

2. Why is a diagnosis so elusive?
Candida symptoms mirror many other conditions. As a result it is often a matter of elimination of other diseases and the knowledge/ skill level of the practitioner to determine the presence of Candida. Since Candida symptoms are so broad in scope, some people may

have only one set of symptoms which can be misleading for the practitioner.

3. *Is it OK to do a Candida cleanse without knowing for sure if a person has Candida?*
I have found many people immediately benefit from changing their diet to the Candida diet. If a person's body does not find the Candida cleanse effective, the person will usually notice one of the following two sets of symptoms:
a. No symptoms. In this case the cleanse is not hurting and the increase of probiotics is probably helpful. Cleansing is always beneficial. The increased probiotic support of a good Candida cleanse will support the gut and be helpful in boosting the overall work of the immune system.
b. Intestinal pain. In this case the cleanse should be immediately stopped. Either an allergic response or a healing crisis has surfaced. The person should seek out professional help before continuing with the cleanse.

CANDIDA SYMPTOMS
GENERAL SYMPTOMS
- ♦ chronic fatigue
- ♦ lack of energy
- ♦ sense of poor well-being

GASTROINTESTINAL SYMPTOMS
- ♦ dry mouth
- ♦ rash or blisters in mouth
- ♦ bad breath
- ♦ thrush (coated tongue)
- ♦ bloating, belching, intestinal gas
- ♦ intestinal cramps
- ♦ heartburn, reflux
- ♦ indigestion
- ♦ rectal itching

- diarrhea
- constipation
- mucus in stools
- hemorrhoids
- IBS (irritable bowel syndrome)
- bread and/or sugar cravings

GENITO-URINARY SYMPTOMS
- vaginal yeast infections
- frequent bladder infections

ENDOCRINE SYMPTOMS
- PMS
- menstrual cramps
- endometriosis
- joint pain or swelling
- prostatitis
- loss of sex drive

LYMPHATIC SYMPTOMS
- post nasal drip
- sinus problems
- nasal itching
- sore or dry throat
- cough
- wheezing or shortness of breath
- ear pain, ringing or deafness
- fluid in the ears
- ear infections

NERVOUS SYSTEM SYMPTOMS
- depression
- irritable
- brain fog
- mood swings
- frequent pains

ORGAN SYMPTOMS
- ◆ toxic liver
- ◆ skin problems (i.e., psoriasis, eczema, hives, blemishes)
- ◆ itching
- ◆ erratic vision
- ◆ spots in front of eyes

IMMUNE SYSTEM SYMPTOMS
- ◆ allergies
- ◆ chemical sensitivities
- ◆ low immune function

CHILDREN'S SYMPTOMS
- ◆ ear infections
- ◆ allergies
- ◆ thrush
- ◆ mom had Candida

CANDIDA SELF ANALYSIS

The following questionaire is available on our website at www.lifestyleforhealth.com.

HISTORY – SECTION 1

This section involves an understanding of your medical history and how it may have promoted Candida growth. Circle those comment to which you can answer *yes*. Record your total at the end of the section.

Points

1. Throughout your lifetime, have you taken any   25
    antibiotics or tetracyclines (Symycin™, Panmycin™,
    Bivramycin™, Monicin™ etc.) for acne or other
    conditions, for more than one month?

Points

2. Have you ever taken a "broad spectrum" antibiotic   20
   for more than two months or four or more times in
   a one-year period? These could include any antibiotics
   taken for respiratory, urinary or other infections.

3. Have you taken a "broad spectrum" antibiotic   6
   — even for a single course? These antibiotics
   include ampicillin™, amoxicillin™, Keflex™, etc.

4. Have you ever had problems with persistent   25
   prostatitis, vaginitis or other problems with
   your reproductive organs?

5. Women — Have you been pregnant:
   Two or more times?   5
   One time?   3

6. Women — Have you taken birth control pills:
   More than two years?   15
   More than six months?   8

7. If you were not breast-fed as an infant.   9

8. Have you taken any cortisone-type drugs   15
   (Prednisone™, Decadron™, etc.)?

9. Are you sensitive to and bothered by exposure
   to perfumes, insecticides or other chemical odors:
   Do you have moderate to severe symptoms?   20
   Do you have mild symptoms?   5

10. Does tobacco smoke bother you?   10

11. Are your symptoms worse on damp, muggy days   20
    or in moldy places?

12. If you have had chronic fungus infections of the
    skin or nails (including athlete's foot, ring worm,
    jock itch), have the infections been:
    Severe or persistent?   20
    Mild to moderate?   10

13.	Do you crave sugar (chocolate, ice cream, candy, cookies, etc.)?	10
14.	Do you crave carbohydrates (bread, bread and more bread)?	10
15.	Do you crave alcoholic beverages?	10
16.	Have you drunk or do you drink chlorinated water (city or tap)?	20

Total Score Section 1 _____

MAJOR SYMPTOMS – SECTION 2

For each of your symptoms, enter the appropriate figure in the point score column.

No symptoms	0
Occasional or mild	3
Frequent and/or moderately severe	6
Severe and/or disabling	9

Points

1.	Constipation	____
2.	Diarrhea	____
3.	Bloating	____
4.	Fatigue or lethargy	____
5.	Feeling drained	____
6.	Poor memory	____
7.	Difficulty focusing/brain fog	____
8.	Feeling moody or despair	____
9.	Numbness, burning or tingling	____

10. Muscle aches   ____

11. Nasal congestion or discharge   ____

12. Pain and/or swelling in the joints   ____

13. Abdominal pain   ____

14. Spots in front of the eyes   ____

15. Erratic vision   ____

16. Cold hands and/or feet   ____

Women

17. Endometriosis   ____

18. Menstrual irregularities and/or severe cramps   ____

19. PMS   ____

20. Vaginal discharge   ____

21. Persistent vaginal burning or itching   ____

Men

22. Prostatitis   ____

23. Impotence   ____

Women and Men

24. Loss of sexual desire   ____

25. Low blood sugar   ____

26. Anger or frustration   ____

27. Dry, patchy skin   ____

Total Score Section 2   _____

MINOR SYMPTOMS – SECTION 3

For each of your symptoms, enter the appropriate figure in the point score column.

No symptoms	0
Occasional or mild	1
Frequent and/or moderately severe	2
Severe and/or disabling	3

Points

1. Heartburn   _____

2. Indigestion   _____

3. Belching and intestinal gas   _____

4. Drowsiness   _____

5. Itching   _____

6. Rashes   _____

7. Irritability or jitters   _____

8. Uncoordinated   _____

9. Inability to concentrate   _____

10. Frequent mood swings   _____

11. Postnasal drip   _____

12. Nasal itching   _____

13. Failing vision   _____

14. Burning or tearing of the eyes   _____

15. Recurrent infections of fluid in the ears   _____

16. Ear pain or deafness   _____

17. Headaches   _____

18. Dizziness/loss of balance _____

19. Pressure above the ears _____
    (your head feels like it is swelling and tingling)

20. Mucus in the stool _____

21. Hemorrhoids _____

22. Dry mouth _____

23. Rash or blisters in the mouth _____

24. Bad breath _____

25. Sore or dry throat _____

26. Cough _____

27. Pain or tightness in the chest _____

28. Wheezing or shortness of breath _____

29. Urinary urgency or frequency _____

30. Burning during urination _____

Total Score Section 3 _____

THE RESULTS

Total Score from Section 1 _____
Total Score from Section 2 _____
Total Score from Section 3 _____

Total Score _____

See the next page to interpret your score.

Total Score from page 61 _____

If your score is at least	*Your symptoms are:*
180 Women	Almost certainly yeast connected
140 Men	Almost certainly yeast connected
120 Women	Probably yeast connected
90 Men	Probably yeast connected
60 Women	Possibly yeast connected
40 Men	Possibly yeast connected

If your score is less than	*Your symptoms are:*
60 Women	Probably not yeast connected
40 Men	Probably not yeast connected

If your score is 60+ (women) or 40+ (men), then you will probably want to consider following the suggestions found in the remainder of this book.

CASE STUDIES

As I share stories of people with whom we have worked, it is important that I remind you that *I am not a doctor. I do not diagnose nor do I prescribe.* My entire approach is to equip a person to identify stressers in his/her body and real and/or imagined stumbling blocks to achieving optimal health.

I am not suggesting that anyone else will achieve the same results as these cases, even if they follow the same protocol. The only reason for sharing these stories is to give hope that there is an answer. I am offended at any health care provider who refuses to give hope to a person who wants to improve their health. Without hope there is no reason to fight or to win ... the health issue is indeed *hopeless!*

BEGIN TO HOPE!

If these stories do nothing but give you hope that there is an answer to your "health opportunity" then I have met my goal. If someone had not extended hope to me in 1990, when my health had completely crashed, I would not be writing this book or helping thousands of others regain their health.

Hope means to:
    have a desire of something good
    have some expectation of that "good thing" happening
    place confidence in something or somebody

Many people *wish for* or *desire* health, but have no real *hope* that health can happen for them. It is important to understand the difference in these three words. Their definitions demonstrate more than mere semantics — they represent significant heart and identify differences.

When a person is *hoping* for a health change, they have a solid reason for that hope and are assured that hope will provide some form of pleasure or joy in the final outcome. When a person is merely *wishing for* or *desiring* a health change, they usually have no reason for the change, are unwilling to actually change much in their life and may easily experience pain and/or anxiety when confronted with any choices.

To confront a health issue with no hope is to have a living death sentence on the installment plan. Hope allows a person to draw on reserves they never knew existed and accomplish more than they ever dreamed possible. That just may be the first step in your success ... to once again have hope that health is a real possibility in your life. To have a hope that is based on solid evidence, willingness to change and a commitment to diligently pursue the goal of health.

TAKE RESPONSIBILITY FOR YOUR HEALTH

As I work with individuals and/or families, I continue to push the responsibility of health back into their hands. The choices are theirs, the consequences are theirs and the victories are theirs. I am a resource, along with hundreds of other team players — health care providers, friends, books and educational resources. The key is to get the entire team pulling for a win instead of each going in a different direction.

(All names have been changed for confidentiality purposes.)

Case #1: Alice

I had known Alice for over nine years. Approximately one year before I began to work with her, I saw her at a birthday party of a mutual friend. Alice looked terrible! She had gained a lot of weight, was puffy and was obviously not feeling well. We talked briefly. She acknowledged she had a problem but was having little success in addressing it.

Shortly thereafter she became engaged. The couple continually delayed the wedding date due to her health. One year after that encounter, she came to one of our conferences. I could hardly believe my eyes — she looked worse. She looked like a sponge ready to explode.

A new boldness had become a part of my lifestyle and I confronted her. "You need to see me or someone and work on this health issue!" I exclaimed. I left it at that. Due to a series of "coincidences, (otherwise known as God-plans), I had an appointment cancellation and she came into my office only five days later.

We tested her and sure enough she showed high levels of stress with Candida. We identified a supplement and dietary plan to reduce her stress load. Within two weeks she began to experience Candida die-off symptoms. She was fatigued, nauseous and had headaches. Alice called me in a state of frustration and weakness. We prayed and I gave her several options. She chose to continue the cleanse. That weekend, after a couple of enemas, she passed several unusual bowels.

The next day, Alice had a breakthrough. From total despair two days ago, she was now feeling good. She went to the local health food store and had another amazing breakthrough: Alice passed the bakery without any sugar cravings! She was ecstatic! The good news continued. Within one month she had lost fifteen pounds, eleven inches and all of her headaches. She had also lost pain she didn't even know she had until it quit hurting! Her skin began to glow and the brain fog was a thing of the past.

Two months into the process she began to experience a few sugar cravings and some body temperature variations. We retested her stress load, made some adjustments and she went to another level of breakthroughs.

Today, Alice and her fiancé (interestingly enough he also had Candida and has begun his cleanse) have set a wedding date and she is thrilled that she has "a life."

What can you learn from Alice? Alice told me, "I had lost all hope. I wasn't sure I would ever get better. Being without hope was the hardest part. If nothing else you gave me hope."

Alice did the work — I have never had a client who read more, studied more or did more. Alice applied what she learned from me, other health care providers and her own reading. She was diligent and consistent. She called when she needed help, but she did what she needed to do. Alice took personal responsibility for her health.

Although I had some expertise and experience, the most valuable service I gave to Alice was *hope*. That *hope* gave her the stamina to continue on until she won. She became "more than a conqueror!"

Case #2: Ron

Ron and his wife came in for testing. The protocol we developed for his wife was producing benefits for her, but nothing seemed to work for Ron. Often I *wished* he would just quit coming in. I could not figure out how to help Ron.

Ron refinished furniture. His body showed high levels of stress on his liver from the toxic load of his job. He had wide mood swings, was constantly fatigued and quite depressed. We tried a variety of cleanses and immune builders. Nothing seemed to work. I had come as close to losing hope as ever with any client. I couldn't get rid of him because he just kept coming back!

One day, out of frustration, I checked Ron for Candida. I had fallen into the trap of thinking Candida primarily hit women. Behold, we had an answer to at least part of his stress — he showed Candida.

I gave him our suggested diet, cleanse and supplement protocol for Candida. I must admit I had little *hope* he would follow through. Sure enough, I saw Ron's name on the calendar four weeks later. Great! I thought. I'll bet that didn't work either.

I was in for a surprise. He had grudgingly made the diet changes (he admitted he was mad at me for suggesting the changes — they were his favorite foods!). He had followed the cleanse and supplement suggestions. He was having emotional and physical breakthroughs and was feeling great for the first time in years!

What can you learn from Ron? Often, you need to hold onto *hope* even when your health care provider has little or no hope. If Ron had followed my example, he would have stopped just short of his breakthrough.

The lesson with Ron did not stop with Ron, it affected me. I learned, once again, to not make assumptions. Candida can impact men, children and women. I was encouraged to be more persistent in working with people, especially the clients who are themselves persistent.

Last but not least, we both learned it was a team process. He continued when I was ready to quit. I was tough when he was ready to quit. He also had a wife who was equally strong in her commitment to his health. Together we became a "team" that made a touchdown. Ron's game of life is not over, but has gained many points and is doing much better!

Case #3: John
John and his family had come in for testing. His wife and children were doing well, however John carried about 25 pounds which he

could not drop. Everything we tried failed. I was discouraged and so was John.

One defeat, however, did not stop John. He kept looking for an answer. One day he was in a health food store and he began to talk to the owner. She suggested he take the Candida Self-test (found in Appendix F). He passed that test with flying colors! He began a Candida cleanse, changed his diet and dropped 25 pounds in one month.

I truly appreciate John. He came back to me and told me of his breakthrough. At that time I was not testing each person on Candida. After I did my homework, I began to regularly test for Candida. As a result of John talking to me, I was able to provide insight for Ron, Alice and literally thousands of other people. Thank you, John, for taking the time to share your success with me and many other people.

What can you learn from John? No one person has all the answers to all the problems of all the people! Anyone who thinks he has all of the answers is in heavy delusion!

When you do not experience a success with one health care provider, keep looking. I firmly believe there is an answer to every problem, if a person knows the right questions to ask and of whom to ask those questions. (By the way that is the Hebrew definition of wisdom!)

I was not the right person for John to ask his questions. He continued to ask and eventually he found a person with the right answers for him. The good news is that John knew my heart was motivated to help others. He took the time to share his answers with me. I learned from John because I want to grow, improve and help more people.

If your health care provider is closed to new information, thinks only she has all of the answers, you might want to move on. Each of us can learn from each other. Health is a partnership ... be sure you plug into a partnership that is based on wisdom, good fruit and healthy communication. Avoid any partnership that is based on ego, stagnant learning and manipulation. You deserve better! Remember, you are paying the bill!

I could share many more stories with you, but these three lay a good foundation. Over and over they show the need for hope, persistence and the need to question. All three cases seemed hopeless, but they weren't. Today they have hope, new fruit and new vision. You, too, can move on.... Renew your hope, persist and learn to ask good questions of wise people.

FOUR
CANDIDA SOLUTIONS
✦✦✦

A fter much research, reading and testing, I have found that the following eight steps must be included in any effective Candida protocol. Leaving out any one of these steps greatly reduces your success and increases your chance of reoccurrence of the Candida problem.

The following will provide you with the specific protocol that I have used on myself, my family and with clients. You will also find helpful recipes in Appendix C to help you implement the Candida diet.

EIGHT STEPS TO ADDRESS CANDIDA

1. Eliminate or minimize the use of antibiotics, steroids, immune-suppressing drugs and birth control pills. *Please be sure to seek the advice of your health care provider before you stop taking any prescriptions.*
2. Make diet changes.
3. Enhance digestion and assimilation.
4. Do a Candida cleanse.
5. Enhance immune function.
6. Enhance healthy bacteria flora.
7. Increase fiber consumption.
8. Maintain to prevent repeated occurrence of Candida!

Let's review each of these steps. Many methods and cleanses can be used, but I have found that the effective programs included each of these steps.

STEP 1 – ELIMINATE USE OF ANTIBIOTICS, STEROIDS, IMMUNE-SUPPRESSING DRUGS AND BIRTH CONTROL PILLS.
If you have taken the History and Symptoms List Questionnaire in Chapter Three, then it should be apparent that these types of prescriptions are the biggest contributors to Candida. Continued use of them will cripple any Candida protocol.

If you are taking antibiotics, steroids or immune-suppressing drugs, work with your health care provider to determine safer options. Realize that the more you do to boost your immune system (see Appendix A) the less you will even need to consider antibiotics. If your health care provider is not aware of any options to antibiotics, seek out a second opinion.

If you are taking prescriptions for your skin, work with your health care provider to determine a safe way to come off of them. Numerous clients who follow the Lifestyle for Health Candida protocol see tremendous improvements in their skin. The skin improvement was made without any use of prescription drugs.

If you are taking birth control pills to regulate your menstrual cycle, once again work with your health care provider to determine a safe way to come off of the pill. I have seen success in cycle-regulation when the correct hormonal and Candida approach was taken. If you are taking birth control pills to prevent pregnancy, consider other options that are healthier for your body. Be sure to check with your health care provider before stopping any prescription drug.

STEP 2 – MAKE DIET CHANGES
Certain foods feed the yeast. Consuming those foods only perpetuates the problem. The clients I have worked with experience a faster relief of symptoms the more they avoid the following foods. However, even if they did not 100% eliminate these foods (only eliminated 30% to 50%), they experienced a level of success.

Some of you are of the obsessive/compulsive order that thinks they must do everything perfectly (that was the old me!) or nothing at all. If you are of that opinion, take note: It is okay to do the best that you can. Moving in the right direction will eventually get you to your destination. It is better to go slower and make it than to drive so hard you kill yourself in the process. This maxim is true in the health arena as much as it is on the road.

If on the other hand you tend to be a little too laid back and think that a "little" of this and a "little" of that won't matter, take note: Unlike the obsessive/compulsive people, your "little" is rarely "little." You must learn to avoid these foods with a "little" more persistence!

Be sure to read labels carefully! You will be surprised how many of these foods are in other packaged foods. For example, vinegar is in ketchup, mustard, mayonnaise and pickles. Don't assume, read the labels!

The foods to avoid include:

- ◆ yeast (i.e., bread and all foods containing yeast)
- ◆ alcohol (especially beer and wine)
- ◆ cheese
- ◆ dried fruits
- ◆ peanuts
- ◆ refined sugar (and all foods containing sugar)
- ◆ natural sweeteners (this includes honey, maple syrup, Sucanat, molasses, etc.)
- ◆ fruit (the only fruit that is recommended is Granny Smith apples)
- ◆ fermented foods (i.e., vinegar, tofu, soy sauce, tamari)
- ◆ dairy (if there is a dairy allergy)
- ◆ wheat (especially if Blood Type is O)
- ◆ all allergenic foods

I'm sure that after you read that list you probably felt you would die since there is nothing left to eat! The problem with most people with Candida is that the above list is what they eat, what they crave and what feeds their problem.

There are actually many foods left to eat and Chapter Five (Candida Diet) will address those foods and how to get them into your daily diet.

STEP 3 – ENHANCE DIGESTION AND ASSIMILATION

Digestive complaints and food allergies are another key link to Candida. Due to the high level of processed foods consumed by people with Candida, there is often a deficiency of enzymes.

Digestion refers to the mechanical and chemical process of breaking down food from large molecules to small molecules. Assimilation (or absorption) refers to the transport of nutrients across membranes of the GI tract into the bloodstream and lymph stream, where eventually they are carried into cells throughout the body for utilization.

A multimillion-dollar industry has evolved to treat such digestive disorders as reflux, heartburn, burping, bloating, gas, constipate, diarrhea, abdominal cramping, bad breath and body odor. These symptoms are not an indication of using the wrong antacids, mouthwash or mints. They are clearly pointing to the toxic load in the body that is a result of poor digestion and/or assimilation as well as other factors (i.e., fatigue, emotional upset, lowered immune function, etc.).

Instead of reaching for the antacids, mouthwash or mints, consider making the following changes to help your body better digest and assimilate food.

Eat a more natural, raw foods diet.

If you increase your intake of raw foods and notice your symptoms increase, you may need to start by lightly steaming your raw foods. Raw foods include vegetables (ideally they would be organic and vine-ripened — but let's just start with vegetables!), fruits (only Granny Smith apples), nuts (soaking overnight increases their digestibility), seeds (sprouting increases their enzyme content) and whole grains (which need to be cooked and/or soaked).

Consider food combining.

Food combining can become very complex and time consuming. The more challenged the digestive/assimilation system is the more food combining needs to be followed. The following guidelines have simplified food combining for me.

1. Combine protein foods with low-starch vegetables (i.e., do not mix meat and potatoes).
2. Combine starch foods with low-starch vegetables (i.e., do combine potatoes with a salad).
3. Combine nuts and seeds with any food group (a few nuts with fruit works well).
4. Eat fruit alone or 20 minutes before other foods or two hours after other foods.
5. Combine lemon, papaya and pineapple with any other food groups.

Reduce stress.

Stress lowers the production of pancreatic enzymes, shuts down digestion and slows elimination. If the stress is emotional, consider finding a counselor to help you work through the emotional issues. If the stress is job related, do a job assessment. Is the job worth your health? Do you want to prematurely retire due to death or retire and find your health is permanently damaged? The right job for you should be a challenge but also provide an equal source of satisfaction. Don't settle for anything else.

One of the subjects taught at the Lifestyle for Health Education Center is *Destiny*. Many people are unaware of their giftings, skills and interests, let alone their destiny. Your destiny is expressed in your profession which is a result of what you "can't not do." For more information on the LFH Facilitator Program for Body by Design, contact the LFH office at 303-794-4477.

Consider taking a digestive enzyme supplement.

If you experience regular bloating, gas, constipation and diarrhea after eating, a digestive enzyme may be helpful to you. Many good brands of enzymes are available on the market. If you have found the right one for you, you should notice a difference within less than a week. If you have not noticed a difference within a week, you probably do not have the right digestive enzyme match for you. Remember, diligence and persistence are often the keys to optimal health.

Appendix A gives you brands that I have found helpful. Remember, as you eliminate Candida, your digestion and assimilation will improve.

Consider a hydrochloric acid supplement.
If you are over the age of 40, you may be deficient in hydrochloric acid. To determine if this is the case with you, it is recommended that you take a 24-hour urine analysis. A qualified health care provider or LFH Coach can help you in taking this type of testing and in the appropriate analysis. If you are deficient in hydrochloric acid, you will need that type of supplement instead of, or even in addition to, digestive enzymes.

Chew and eat slowly.
One of the most common causes of poor digestion is eating too fast and only gulping food. To digest properly, food must be thoroughly chewed before swallowing. In addition to chewing thoroughly, avoid any sizable consumption of fluids during meals. The more you drink while eating, the more you wash away the first digestive aids in the saliva. It is best to drink before meals or an hour or two after your meal.

Consider juicing.
Consuming freshly made juices can greatly increase the presence of digestive enzymes. Raw fruits and vegetables are rich in enzymes, which are the sparks for digestion to occur. However, in the presence of Candida, carrot juice can add to the problem as carrots are naturally high in sugar. It is better to juice greens. Since they are so bitter, a few Granny Smith apples can be included to improve taste.

STEP 4 – CANDIDA CLEANSE

A cleanse is the most aggressive way to eliminate the Candida problem. I highly recommend the Candida cleanse. The next chapter will go into more detail on the Candida cleanses which I use. Whatever protocol you choose to use, you want to be sure it includes a cleanse.

A good Candida cleanse should have the following elements:

1. Probiotics
Probiotics are essential for the GI tract to begin to restore natural flora balance. Without good probiotics, any Candida cleanse is incomplete. Both acidophilus and bifidum are needed in some form. These probiotics must be in a live, stable format so that they can actually recolonize in the gut.

Providing saccharide support (either from fructoligosaccharides or glyconutrients which can contain up to eight saccharides) helps the probiotics multiply faster. Both the cleanse and the maintenance program that I recommend include probiotics and saccharide support.

2. Zinc tannates
Tannates are powerful, natural substances that bind to bad bacteria and fungus in your body rendering them ineffective.

3. Pau d'arco bark
Pau d'arco is a recognized herb that is effective in battling Candida. It should be found in either the cleanse product and/or in tea that is consumed throughout the day. Pau d'arco made into tea can also be used in enemas for further cleansing.

4. Garlic
One of the top five immune builders (according to Dr. Darryl See) is garlic.[1] Garlic should be an ingredient in the cleanse product and/or added as a supplement and/or used in enemas to aggressively fight the Candida.

Other cleanses

In addition to the Candida cleanse, several other types of cleanses should be considered.

Emotional cleansing is important. Control, fear and/or anger can greatly impact the functioning of the bowel and skin. If those emotions are not handled, any Candida cleanse will be limited.

Exercise helps. The lymphatic system must be able to handle the detox process, so anything that supports the lymph improves the success rate of a Candida cleanse. Exercise helps stimulate the lymphatic system and is also helpful in resolving stress and some emotional buildup. Using rebounders (miniature trampolines) and walking are especially helpful in this area.

Skin brushing also helps stimulate the lymph flow. Natural bristle brushes can be purchased from Lifestyle for Health (see order form) or from health food stores. Before starting to dry brush the skin, stimulate the two primary lymph ducts. These ducts can be found at the base of the collar bone (one on each side) and also in the groin area. Rub these areas for a few seconds to get the ducts opened. To skin brush effectively, follow this procedure and brush three to six times a week:

1. Open ducts (to do this gently massage just below the collar bone — 1 set of ducts — and in the groin area — 2nd set of ducts.
2. Brush dry skin with clean, frequently washed natural bristle brush.
3. Use small, light circular motions.
4. Start close to the ducts and work outward.
5. From the waist up, brush toward the upper pair of ducts (under collar bone).
6. From the waist down, brush toward the lower pair of ducts (in groin area).

Liver cleanse. A person with Candida often has a sluggish liver. Cleansing the liver can help restore liver function. An aggressive liver cleanse is not recommended to be done at the same time as a Candida cleanse unless you are under the supervision of a qualified health care provider. However, after a Candida cleanse you may want to consider a liver cleanse.

Parasite cleanse. Some people who have Candida also have parasites. I usually recommend a parasite cleanse following a Candida cleanse. Parasite testing can be done by health care providers to ensure their presence. Ann Louise Gittleman has an excellent book, *Guess What Came to Dinner,* that discusses parasites and how to do a parasite cleanse.

Several good parasite cleanses exist, both herbal and homeopathic. Appendix A gives you the brands that I have found to be effective.

STEP 5 – ENHANCE IMMUNE FUNCTION

Obviously it is important to improve the immune function when fighting Candida. Improved immune function must include the lymphatic system. The lymphatic system is the one area that I find that many health care providers overlook in Candida cleanses.

Without effective lymphatic system support, people can feel terrible before they get better. In fact, some people may never be able to see improvement because their discomfort overrides their very real desire to pursue the cleanse. Their body may be unable to handle the detoxification process due to a poorly functioning lymphatic system.

The lymphatic system pulls metabolic waste from body tissues, processes these toxins through the nodes and sends them out various detox pathways. These pathways include the lungs, skin, colon and kidneys. When any of these pathways are sluggish or shut down, then the other pathways have an extra burden to carry. In time, each pathway can become sluggish or ineffective and then the lymphatic system is hindered. At this point any cleanse can produce serious consequences.

Few health care providers do much with the lymphatic system. When it is addressed, often only herbs (i.e., echinacea) are used. I have found that herbal support alone is usually not enough to get the lymphatic system freely moving.

In my work I have found that homeopathic lymph support can be quite effective. Testing a client for lymph support is essential as there are many lymph homeopathics. Sometimes the client has excess mucus that must be dissolved. Some clients lack adequate lymph drainage but have no mucus buildup.

Knowing which lymphatic support remedy to use is as important as knowing that one is needed. Concentrated homeopathic lymph support should be provided by qualified health care providers. General homeopathic lymph remedies are listed in Appendix A. I also recommend skin brushing, exercise, massage and deep breathing to stimulate the lymphatic system.

The lymphatic system is impacted by suppressed emotions. I often term the lymph a symbol of "unshed tears." During the time the lymphatic system is supported, it is common for emotional issues to surface.

In addition to supporting the lymphatic system, the rest of the immune system needs to be built up. Up to 70% of American adults use some form of dietary supplement to improve immune function. However, despite expenditures on these supplements increasing each year, only a few of these products have scientific proof of their efficacy in restoring or maintaining health (i.e., the immune function). Furthermore, the toxicity of these products has rarely been studied. To improve overall health, any supplement intended for immune enhancement must be nontoxic and beneficial.

Dr. Darryl See is a leading researcher in the area of immune system support and the former associate Clinical Professor of Medicine in the Division of Infectious Diseases at UC Irvine Medical School. He has received two National Institute of Health research grants and has rigorously pursued the issue of immune function. Dr. See decided to study supplements and their impact on the immune system. The results of Dr. See's research can be found in the 1999 Winter Edition of the *Journal of the American Nutraceutical Association* (JANA).[2] You can obtain a copy of JANA by contacting the Lifestyle for Health office at 303-794-4477.

The purpose of his study was to screen commonly used dietary supplements that claim to have immune enhancing, antioxidant or broad anti-microbial activity. The supplements were screened for toxicity, NK cell function, intracellular glutathione (GSH) augmentation, antiviral activity and cytochrome modulation (liver enzyme function). These parameters were chosen as they are particularly important in the health of cells, which may translate to improvement or maintenance in the general health of the consumer. His study showed:

♦ Nearly 50% of the products tested were toxic.
♦ 42.5% of the products impacted cytochrome activity (i.e., interference of liver metabolism).
♦ Glyconutrient-containing products had significant NK enhancing effect.
♦ Five products were found to be non-toxic, without cytochrome effect and had a significant effect on the three efficacy tests.

The number one product, based on overall effectiveness and least toxicity, was a complex naturally occurring plant polysaccharide (a glyconutrient). The next four products included two products containing glyconutrients, along with aloe vera and garlic. Recommendations for these supplements are provided in Appendix A.

STEP 6 – ENHANCE HEALTHY BACTERIA FLORA

As I have already mentioned, healthy bacteria (probiotics) are a crucial ingredient for any effective Candida cleanse. This is true not only during the cleanse but after the cleanse. The natural way to get probiotics is in yogurt.

Yogurt is not the probiotic-dead, sugar-filled, additive-pumped stuff found on the shelves of most grocery stores! I use plain yogurt made with live cultures from antibiotic-free milk. This would include brands such as Horizon, Cascadian Farms, Nancy, etc.

However, if a person is sensitive to yogurt, this option may not work. Most people can benefit from a probiotic supplement both during and after a cleanse. Appendix A gives brands I have found to be effective.

STEP 7 – INCREASE FIBER

If you are the average American who has consumed the Standard American Diet (SAD!!!), then you are sure to have a fiber deficiency. Without enough fiber, the body is unable to effectively cleanse the colon and effectively absorb essential nutrients.

Fiber is important in lowering blood cholesterol levels and stabilizing blood sugar levels. It is also helpful in removing toxins from the body including heavy metals. There are seven basic classifications of fiber: bran, cellulose, gum, hemicellulose, lignin, mucilages and pectin. Each form has a benefit and it is best to rotate among several different supplement sources.

It is crucial to take fiber supplements at least 30 minutes away from other supplements and any medications!

Fiber can also be added through dietary changes. Include high-fiber foods, such as whole grain flours, brown rice, fresh fruits, nuts, seeds (especially flax), beans, lentils and fresh vegetables. When consuming fiber be sure to drink enough water to prevent bloating.

STEP 8 – MAINTENANCE PROGRAM

At a recent seminar I gave on Candida, a woman came by to tell me her story. She had done a rigorous Candida cleanse by closely following all of the above steps while working with another health care provider. She closely followed each step for over six months and had experienced much improvement. After that period she stopped the protocol and was not placed on a maintenance program. Within less than one month, she was back to craving sugar and bread and many of her old symptoms had returned!

I'm not sure which is worse: not doing a cleanse or doing one and not doing a maintenance plan. I shudder to think of the frustration of diligently following a Candida diet, experiencing success and then ending up back at square one because no maintenance was put into place.

The maintenance plan that I have found effective is given in the next chapter. This is my own personal maintenance plan. I may add to it to work on specific issues, but I never do less than it.

Whoops, I must admit that one month I took a break from this plan. I decided I had been eating healthy and taking supplements for nearly ten years, I "deserved" a break from the rigors. Of course this occurred during the month of December! Before long I was eating more of my "healthier" sweets. I noticed my hair wasn't growing very fast (I usually need a haircut every three weeks!) and it was beginning to fall out. I wanted more of my "good home-made breads."

It wasn't long until my lightning-quick brain figured out I had the signs of Candida. I had a live blood cell analysis done and sure enough ... I had more of those critters than I wanted! I began the Candida cleanse (presented in the next chapter) and began to experience improvement in a matter of two weeks.

Once again, I know how important a *lifestyle* of health is. A lifestyle is an all-the-time, not part-time process. Likewise, eliminating Candida is not just a one-time cleanse process ... it is an on-going lifestyle. No truer words were ever spoken than:

"Health — It's a Lifestyle!"

NOTES FOR CHAPTER FOUR

1. Darryl See, Ph.D., *Journal of the American Nutraceutical Association (JANA)*, Winter, 1999, vol. 2, no. 1.

2. Ibid.

FIVE
CANDIDA CLEANSE ...
THE LFH PROTOCOL
♦♦♦

When I work with someone who shows the presence of Candida, whether through the use of the questionnaire, biofeedback or blood work, I work with some variation of the following Lifestyle for Health protocol. It is important that you work with a qualified health care provider in developing your Candida program.

The following suggested protocol is not meant to diagnose, prescribe or be used for therapeutic measures.

I am not a paid spokesperson for any of the products that I recommend. Though it is certainly acceptable for folks to be paid spokespeople for companies, I found out the hard way that it limits my objectivity and freedom to honestly recommend what is truly best. As I make product recommendations throughout this book, please keep in mind that these recommendations are based on the way the products work with my clients, our readers and myself.

CANDIDA CLEANSES

I have recommended various products over the years for Candida. Unfortunately, some of those products have not maintained the standards I like to see in a product. Over the past couple of years, I have changed my recommendations in this area.

Although the common contributors to Candida are discussed in chapter two, I have found that blood type also plays a significant

---

role in how I go about identifying the appropriate, cleanse. The following overview is not meant to diagnose or prescribe any cure. It is insight based on my clinical experience in working with thousands of clients.

During a detox process, two phases must be covered. First the toxins must be released, which is the cleansing phase. Second, the toxins load must be drained out of the body through detox pathways (colon, lung, bladder and skin). This is the drainage phase. When the drainage phase is omitted, people will experience healing crisis. This may take the form of extreme fatigue, skin rashes, fevers, constipation, wheezing, etc.

Ensuring good drainage with a Candida (or any cleanse) helps reduce these symptoms and facilitate a more comfortable cleanse. Be sure to drink enough water and to exercise. The rebounder continues to be one of the best forms of exercise, especially during a cleanse period.

BLOOD TYPE O

Frequently I see blood type O's having stress in the lung and liver areas. When Candida symptoms show up in O's, I will usually look at a chemical contribution and/or mercury exposure. If this is the case, then the cleanse revolves around a liver cleanse and a lymphatic and/or liver drainer. In addition a probiotic is included.

To determine if enzyme therapy could be helpful, we have the client take our enzyme questionnaire (developed by Dr. Howard Loomis). This questionnaire, available on our website, is a quick easy way for a person to determine which enzyme activity should be supported during a cleanse.

The following protocol has successfully worked with many of the blood type O clients for whom I have worked. Recommended brand names can be found in Appendix A.

1. Probiotic
2. Homeopathic or Herbal Liver Cleanse
   Be sure bowels are moving with 2 – 3 bowel movements a day. If not, do a colon cleanse before the liver cleanse.

3. Homeopathic Drainage
   I find that homeopathics provide excellent drainage during this type of cleanse. I usually ensure drainage of lungs, liver, skin and/or the brain for O's.
4. Essential Fatty Acids
   Flaxseed oil is used to support the skin and circulation.
5. Enzyme Therapy
   The person completes our Enzyme Questionnaire and is tested for the appropriate enzymes. This ensures that digestion, assimilation, cleansing and elimination occur during the cleanse.
6. Candida Diet
   Be sure to have the person avoid wheat, allergenic grains, sugar and dairy.

BLOOD TYPE A

Candida is probably one of the most common problems for a blood type A. The tendency of an A to be overly mental and to have trouble with digestion requires a different approach to the problem. To support these clients, I focus on a more general Candida cleanse (herbal), with extra enzyme and emotional support.

A blood type A must follow the Candida diet more closely than the blood type O. Since digestion tends to be a key issue, keeping food stressors to a minimum speeds the cleansing process.

Emotional stress, (stuffed emotions) also aggravates the Candida issue in an A. The Candida emotional root is a sense of being "out of control" (covered in my book *Discovering Wholeness*). Helping the person recognizes where and why they feel out of control helps reduce stress and encourage the healing process.

The following protocol has successfully worked with many of the blood type O clients for whom I have worked. Recommended brand names can be found in Appendix A.

1. Probiotic
2. Enzyme Therapy
   The person completes our Enzyme Questionnaire (also

available on our website) and is tested for the appropriate enzymes. This ensures that digestion, assimilation, cleansing and elimination occur during the cleanse.

3. Herbal Cleanse
   Herbs included in this cleanse should include: garlic, pau d'arco root, barberry root, oregano, clove and olive leaf. Each of these exhibits therapeutic benefits that help balance fungal growth.

4. Emotional Support
   The person completes our Emotional Questionnaire (also available on our website) to determine the appropriate flower essence support. Usually a customized blend is prepared to help support the emotions during the cleanse.

5. Essential Fatty Acids
   Flaxseed oil is used to support the skin and circulation.

6. Candida Diet
   Closely follow the entire diet.

BLOOD TYPE B

Rarely do I see a B with Candida, unless they have had numerous surgeries, mercury fillings and/or antibiotics. Before testing them for a Candida protocol, I will test them for parasites, which is a more common problem for the B's. More often they will test better for the parasite cleanse. The rest of their cleanses will more closely reflect a blood type O.

The following protocol has successfully worked with many of the blood type O clients for whom I have worked. Recommended brand names can be found in Appendix A.

1. Check for Parasites, First.
   If parasites test positive, do a parasite cleanse.

2. Probiotic

3. Homeopathic Drainage
   I find that homeopathics provide excellent drainage during this type of cleanse. I usually ensure drainage of brain, bladder, liver and/or skin for O's.

4. Essential Fatty Acids
   Flaxseed oil is used to support the skin and circulation.
5. Enzyme Therapy
   The person completes our Enzyme Questionnaire and is tested for the appropriate enzymes. This ensures that digestion, assimilation, cleansing and elimination occur during the cleanse.
6. Diet
   Have the client be sure to omit corn, sugar, mushrooms, dairy and vinegar.

BLOOD TYPE AB

Since AB is the rarest blood type, I see fewer of them than the other types. I find they tend to be more similar to the blood type A's. Since hormone and immune stress are their areas of weakness, I am careful to build the immune function before, during and after a cleanse.

1. Immune Support
   I usually test for glyconutrients, colostrum, garlic and/or green powder support.
2. Probiotic
3. Enzyme Therapy
   The person completes our Enzyme Questionnaire (also available on our website) and is tested for the appropriate enzymes. This ensures that digestion, assimilation, cleansing and elimination occur during the cleanse.
4. Herbal Cleanse
   Herbs included in this cleanse should include: garlic, pau d'arco root, barberry root, oregano, clove and olive leaf. Each of these exhibits therapeutic benefits that help balance out fungal growth.
5. Emotional Support
   The person completes our Emotional Questionnaire (also available on our website) to determine the appropriate flower essence support for them. Usually a customized

blend is prepared to help support the emotions during the cleanse.

6. Essential Fatty Acids
   Flaxseed oil is used to support the skin and circulation.
7. Candida Diet
   Closely follow the entire diet.

LYMPH SUPPORT

As I have mentioned before, I find supporting the lymphatic system during a cleanse critical. In most cases I find that people fit into one of the following categories in their need for lymphatic support.

1. EXCESS MUCUS.

This person has excess levels of mucus that will manifest in one or more of the following symptoms:

   ♦ sinus headaches, infection or pressure
   ♦ ear infections, ringing or partial deafness
   ♦ asthma or bronchial problems
   ♦ mucus in the bowel or urine

This person needs some type of mucus dissolver to help reduce the excess mucus. See Appendix A for recommendations.

2. LYMPH DRAINAGE.

This person tends to have trouble draining the lymphatic fluid and can have the following symptoms:

   ♦ puffiness in the face or throughout the body
   ♦ post nasal drip
   ♦ dry or watery eyes
   ♦ allergic reactions

This person needs some type of lymphatic drainage support. See Appendix A for recommendations.

When taking lymphatic homeopathic support remedies, it is essential to follow good homeopathic protocol. Lifestyle for Health sends a list of guidelines when you order from us. A summary of the key guidelines includes:

♦ Remedies are put under the tongue (sublingual) with no food or drink being added to the mouth for fifteen minutes before or after the recommended dosage.
♦ Most remedies should be held under the tongue for approximately ten seconds before swallowing.
♦ Nicotine and caffeine (coffee, soda, chocolate and black teas) should be avoided as they inhibit absorption.
♦ Mint (i.e., toothpaste, mouthwash, mints, etc.) should be avoided while taking a remedy.
♦ Maintain purified water intake for maximum benefit.

RECOMMENDED DIET

In Chapter Four I mentioned all of the foods to avoid, which for many people may seem like their entire diet. To review, the foods to be avoided include:

♦ yeast (i.e., bread and all foods containing yeast)
♦ alcohol (especially beer and wine)
♦ cheese
♦ dried fruits
♦ peanuts
♦ refined sugar (and all foods containing sugar)
♦ natural sweeteners (this includes honey, maple syrup, Sucanat, molasses, etc.)
♦ fruit (the only fruit that is recommended is Granny Smith apples)
♦ fermented foods (i.e., vinegar, tofu, soy sauce, tamari)
♦ dairy (if there is a dairy allergy)
♦ wheat (especially if Blood Type is O)
♦ any known, personal allergenic foods (common allergenic

foods include: wheat, dairy, soy, eggs, peanuts, citrus and corn)

Each of these foods plays a part in adding to the problem — more Candida — instead of eliminating the problem.

So what does that leave for you to eat? The following recommendation has worked for many of our clients and is actually the basis of a wholesome diet. When the Candida cleanse is finished, more fruit can be added. Here is the diet I recommend.

Vegetables

A serving of green salad (not iceberg lettuce!) each day is very important. I also recommend that people stay away from or at least minimize intake of the starch vegetables, such as corn, potatoes, sweet potatoes and peas.

Experiment with new vegetables, such as jicima (wonderful with guacamole and in a stir fry), asparagus, leeks (great in soups and a stir fry) and kale. In order to stick with this diet, it is important to get beyond the basics of corn, peas and green beans. The produce section of a good health food store can provide a wealth of vegetable options. It is up to you to experiment and develop your tastes to enjoy this variety.

Grains

The recommended whole grains include brown rice (minimal as it is "sweet" in comparison to the other grains), wild rice, quinoa, millet, buckwheat and amaranth.

Many of you may be unfamiliar with some of these grains. Here is a brief description of each one and how to use them.

Quinoa: Traditionally grown in the Andes, the quinoa plant bears tan-colored grains about the size of sesame seeds. Quinoa is similar to amaranth nutritionally (high protein), but it yields a fluffier texture with a distinct flavor. Quinoa cooks quickly (15 minutes) and is an excellent substitution for any brown rice recipe.

Millet: Millet was a staple food in many countries before the use of rice. Millet is the only grain that is not acid in the body and is highly recommended by most nutritionists for allergy diets. It has a high quality protein and is rich in calcium, iron and potassium. It is also very easy to digest. It is often used as a morning cereal, in soups, stews, casseroles, stuffing or puddings.

Buckwheat: Buckwheat is not related to wheat as it is a grass. Buckwheat groats are most often used as the basis for kasha. The buckwheat flour is stronger in flavor than many other flours as the groats have usually been toasted (hence the darker color). A lighter buckwheat flour can be made by putting untoasted buckwheat groats into a blender or flour mill and grinding to a flour texture.

Amaranth: This poppy-seed-sized grain, a botanical cousin to quinoa, was a revered crop of the ancient Incas and Aztecs. It has a nutty and somewhat sweet flavor. It works best where a cohesive texture is desired as in spoon breads, casseroles or hot cereals. Raw amaranth is a nice addition to cornbread and muffins for added texture.

Protein

Sources of protein can vary based on metabolic profile and blood type. In my book *The Food Puzzle,* I lay out the best sources of protein and the best ratios of protein to carbohydrates and fats. Following a customized plan for protein ensures a better cleanse.

If a person is experiencing any digestive complaints (reflux, bloating, gas, constipation and/or diarrhea), then we use our enzyme therapy to increase digestion during the cleanse. Again, the Enzyme Questionnaire is available on our website at no charge.

If you choose to eat meat or poultry, I highly recommend that they come from organic or natural sources. For beef I recommend Coleman in Colorado and Belle Brook Farms in Texas. For poultry I recommend Shelton from California and Rocky Junior in Colorado. Other sources are available in different regions.

The key in purchasing meat or poultry is to know that it is raised without antibiotics, hormones and steroids. Also check into how it is processed. Some poultry is dipped into various preservatives during processing. The cleaner the source, the cleaner the product, the cleaner the you.

Farm fresh, fertile eggs are an excellent source of protein, unless there is an allergy. I have used our biofeedback machine to test people on commercial eggs and fresh eggs. One would test weak (that would be the commercial!) and the fresh eggs would test fine. Once again, the closer the food is to a natural, clean source, the better it is for you.

Other sources of protein that are easy on the budget include beans, lentils and legumes. These protein sources, especially when combined with whole grains, provide a complete protein at an inexpensive price.

Cooked beans can be used in soups, on salads and made into great dips. Beans, such as white beans, can be ground into flour in a blender and used to quickly thicken soups. If you have trouble digesting beans, try the following method:

1. Soak beans overnight or up to 24 hours (this starts the sprouting process).
2. Drain water.
3. Add fresh water and cook the beans with a strip of kombu.

Kombu is a seaweed that is rich in minerals. It also softens the beans and aids in their digestibility. It is the least flavored of the seaweeds (having virtually no taste) and it will dissolve into the beans. It can be removed after cooking the beans, although it usually has dissolved to the point where it is not noticeable. Be sure to omit salt and tomatoes during this first phase of cooking as they will keep the beans from ever softening.

Beans and lentils can also be sprouted. Sprouts are an excellent source of enzymes, which are also good for the digestive system. Be sure the beans and/or lentils are able to sprout and are not a hybrid which will not sprout.

Fish is an excellent source of protein and especially good for people of northern European descent. Be sure the fish is free of parasites. A thorough visual examination will usually reveal the larger parasites.

Nuts and seeds are good sources of protein. They are also excellent sources of good fats. Avoid peanuts as they often have mold and are actually not in the nut family at all. Almonds digest well, are high in calcium and low in fat. Sesame seeds are also high in calcium and rich in protein. Nut and seed butters are good sources of protein and good bases for dips and dressings.

Although tofu and tempeh are good sources of protein, they are also fermented. Avoid them during a Candida cleanse. Many people are surprised to learn that dark green leafy vegetables are also rich in protein. A daily salad of dark, leafy greens goes a long way in providing you with your daily nutritional needs.

Good Fats

Nuts and seeds have already been mentioned. Be careful not to eat too many of these as they do have a high fat content. Avocados are also a rich source of the good fats and help with satiety (food satisfaction).

Butter is far better than margarine which should be avoided at all times. If butter is not desired due to the dairy content, then olive oil can be used. Spectrum has a spun canola oil spread that can also replace butter.

My favorite oil is flaxseed oil. You do not cook with it, but it is an excellent addition to many recipes. Flax is rich in essential fatty acids which are crucial for overall health, especially for a person with Candida. Without a doubt my favorite flax oil (it tests the best and tastes the best!) is Barlean's. Usually one to two tablespoons of flaxseed oil per day is adequate for the average adult (less for children).

Additional Supplements

In addition to the cleanse and diet, several other supplements can be helpful. I usually include protein powder and flaxseed oil in a smoothie. The smoothie is my breakfast standby. It also becomes a great base for most of my supplements on a maintenance program. Specific brands for additional supplements are given in Appendix A. The smoothie recipe I use during a Candida cleanse is:

Candida Cleanse Fruit Smoothie
Makes 1 smoothie for an adult (enough for 2 children). During travel, the basic smoothie can be placed in a shaker and shook.
1 – 1½ cups liquid (water, almond milk, rice milk, soy milk or fruit juice)
½ banana (optional)
¼ – ½ cup fresh or frozen fruit
ice
Cell Essentials™
optional additions

Blend in blender.

Cell Essentials™
1 – 2 scoops of protein powder
1 – 2 tablespoon of flaxseed oil (recommend Barlean's Flaxseed oil)
¼ – ½ teaspoon of glyconutrients (recommend Ambrotose™ by Mannatech)

Optional Ingredients
10 – 20 drops of Trace Minerals ConcenTrace Drops
1 – 3 teaspoons of a green powder
1 teaspoon of colostrum

Change the liquid source and fruits for variety and flavor. Learn to make a smoothie in such a way that you enjoy it. It can be delicious and great for you!

ENEMAS AND COLONICS
Since the colon can be impacted with mucus and is a breeding ground for Candida, people often find that enemas and/or colonics can help ease abdominal discomfort.

Enemas are easy to do and the equipment is inexpensive. Enema bags can be purchased in local pharmacies. It is best to use purified or distilled water. The following procedure can be used for giving an enema.

1. Be sure the tubing is clamped shut.
2. Place the water or diluted tea into the clean enema bag. A total of four cups should be used. Use liquid at room temperature.
3. Hang the bag at waist level. Lie on floor.
4. Insert the enema nozzle (can be lubricated with aloe vera or vitamin E but not petroleum products) into the rectum.
5. Release the clamp and let about half of the fluid flow in.
6. If possible, retain the liquid for ten minutes, lying on the right side. In the beginning most people cannot hold the liquid that long. Do not make yourself uncomfortable.
7. Reclamp the tube, remove the nozzle and empty the bowel into the toilet. Repeat the process with remaining half of enema.

During a Candida cleanse either plain water and/or a pau d'arco tea enema can help relieve abdominal cramping. To make a pau d'arco enema, make one cup of pau d'arco tea according to directions. Dilute it with three cups of purified water and be sure it is not too hot. Follow the directions above.

Colonics can also be helpful. Colonics use about five gallons of water. They can be done professionally (which is recommended for the novice) and then done at home with the use of colema boards. It is best to use filtered and ozonated (added oxygen) for the water. For information on colema boards, see Appendix B.

When doing enemas or colonics it is important to monitor mineral and probiotic levels. It is often best to increase the consumption of both.

COFFEE ENEMAS

Coffee enemas are considered by many to be one of the best liver cleansers. A coffee enema is a low-volume cleanse that helps detox in many ways. It helps to speed up the bowel's emptying process, which makes the detox process occur more quickly. It also helps the liver empty toxins found in the bile ducts. Coffee enemas do not wash out minerals and electrolytes, which are absorbed higher in the bowel. Do not do coffee enemas if gallstones are present.

People sensitive to coffee are often reluctant to try coffee enemas. Since the coffee stays in the sigmoid colon and the caffeine only goes into the liver circulatory system, it is usually safe to use. Consult with your health care provider and use organic coffee. Not knowing the decaf process, I do not recommend using decaf coffee.

To do a coffee enema, heat one quart of purified water to a boil. Add two flat tablespoons of organic coffee and boil for five minutes. Turn off heat. Cool to a lukewarm temperature. Strain out the coffee grounds.

Place the strained coffee liquid into an enema bag. Be sure the tubing is clamped shut. Hang the enema bag at waist level. Hanging the bag too high will force the fluid too high into the intestine. Lie on a covered floor. Insert the enema nozzle, which may be lubricated if needed. Release the clamp and let about half of the coffee flow in. If possible, retain the enema for 10 minutes. After that time period (or sooner, if needed), reclamp the tube, remove the nozzle and empty the bowels into the toilet. Repeat process with remaining half of enema.

LIVER SUPPORT

Often, when Candida is present (especially in blood type O's), support of the liver can be helpful. The following two methods are gentle cleansers and are excellent ways to begin liver support. A full liver cleanse should be done under the supervision of a knowledgeable health practitioner.

LIVER MASSAGE

Lying on the back, use fingertips and gently massage the liver area. The liver can be found by placing your right hand at the base of your right rib cage. Massage in a clockwise circular motion for three to five minutes at a time, two to three times per day.

LIVER PACK

Saturate a white cloth (i.e., wash cloth) with caster oil (can be found in local grocery store). Place on the liver area. Cover with a towel or something to protect clothing. Get in a comfortable position (i.e., sitting in bed or chair). Rest in this position for 45 minutes. When finished, wash off the oil. It is best to do a pack in the evening as you may feel tired when finished. Liver packs can be done up to every other day or less as needed. For more information, contact a LFH coach.

CANDIDA DIE-OFF SYMPTOMS

During a Candida cleanse, some people may experience Candida die-off symptoms as they increase their intake of the herbs. These symptoms, if they occur, will usually occur in the second or third week. These die-off symptoms include:

- ◆ headaches
- ◆ nausea
- ◆ brain fog
- ◆ dizziness
- ◆ fatigue
- ◆ sugar cravings
- ◆ minor skin breakouts
- ◆ cold hands and feet

A person experiencing these symptoms is usually quite toxic. The symptoms are temporary and can last from a couple of days up to two weeks. If they are too uncomfortable, reduce the dosage of cleanse tablets. If they persist, stop and see your health care provider. Enemas and colonics can help diminish these symptoms.

SIX
AFTER CANDIDA
✦✦✦

If you do not follow a good maintenance plan after completing a Candida cleanse, it is very likely you will repeat the occurrence of Candida. I have found that some people feel so good on the cleanse they choose to eat a modified Candida diet and continue the cleanse for several months. I personally have benefited from doing that for several months at a time.

When the Candida cleanse is complete (determined by you and/or your health care provider), then it is essential to immediately start a maintenance program. Each person is unique so a customized plan is best. However, I have found that most people benefit from at least using the supplements detailed under "Maintenance Plan" in this chapter. I personally use these and a few more to maintain optimal health. Specific brand recommendations can be found in Appendix A.

WHEN TO STOP A CLEANSE

Debbie (different name) attended one of my *Destroy Candida* seminars. She had followed a rigorous Candida diet, cleanse and parasite cleanse for six months. She felt she was done and went off of the cleanse. Within days the sugar and bread cravings were back. She was at this point when she attended the seminar. "What's wrong?" she asked.

Debbie had a problem common to many people. They do the hard work — the diet changes, colonics, a cleanse and take supplements — in a very aggressive manner. Then when they stop the cleanse and begin to add the eliminated foods back into their diet, they revert back to square one.

In many cases this is due to no maintenance plan being put into effect. When testing Debbie we found that she needed additional enzyme support and a glyconutrient support to boost her immune system's ability to keep the Candida albicans in balance. We also found she did better on a different essential fatty acid. Recommendations for these products can be found in Appendix A.

Don't go to all of the trouble of doing a Candida cleanse without planning a maintenance program and some ongoing lifestyle changes. If a person does the cleanse, changes her diet and still finds she has lost minimal weight, I suggest she consider testing for hypoglycemia and/or diabetes. The pancreas/stomach may need some support. It is also important to consider the presence of parasites and to do a parasite cleanse.

PARASITE CLEANSES

The Centers for Disease Control found that over 900,000 people become sick in the U.S. each year from water contaminated with biological organisms.[1] Parasites cause more human devastation and kill more people worldwide than does cancer.[2] In his *The Detox Book*, Dr. Fife states that health experts believe that 80% of Westerners are affected with some type of parasite.[3]

Tests do not always detect their presence. Labs test for only 40 or 50 of the thousands of types of parasites that can live in the body. Most tests are performed on stool samples and some parasites do not reside in the digestive tract.

Parasites come from many sources. They can come from the air, contaminated bedding, pets, handling raw meat and through international travel. Water, especially tap water, is one of the most common sources of parasites. Chlorination of today's water has eliminated the plagues of cholera and typhoid that were common at the turn of the century. Chlorine-resistant organisms, however, can be quite dangerous in our water supply. These organisms include viruses, bacteria, protozoan, amoebas and parasites.

Parasite invasions can manifest in a host of symptoms. Parasites are often found in people with Candida. An effective herbal parasite cleanse must contain three herbs: black walnut, wormwood (also known as Artemesia) and cloves. The walnut and wormwood kill the adults and the cloves kill the eggs. With most herbal parasite cleanses, it is helpful to follow the protocol for two weeks, take off for five days and repeat the cycle. Herbal parasite cleanses are most effective and the most expensive.

Another type of parasite cleanse is a homeopathic. These parasite cleanses work about 75% of the time, are much less expensive and easier for people who have trouble swallowing large quantities of pills.

I have found parasites are so common that I personally do a parasite cleanse every year. Children are more susceptible to parasites — look at all that goes into their mouths!. Teens can usually do adult dosages unless they are very small or light-weight. There are rarely any side effects to these cleanses and they can usually be taken with other medications and supplements.

For recommendations of either type of parasite cleanse, please see Appendix A.

WHEAT INTOLERANCES

Wheat sensitivities are common in people with blood types O and A. Wheat is one of the most common allergies. During a Candida cleanse I usually suggest people avoid wheat as much as possible.

In some people the sensitivity is not just to wheat, it is to all grains containing gluten. Gluten intolerance, also known as Celiac Sprue, can also impact people with Candida. Gluten is the sticky substance in grains that interacts with yeast to provide the structure for bread.

Some people with gluten intolerance can have "sticky stools." If a person has a difficult time cleaning himself after a bowel movement, it can be undigested gluten. Avoiding gluten in all of its forms will almost immediately help this symptom.

Another common symptom of gluten intolerance is rectal bleeding. I have seen clients experience an almost complete stop in profuse rectal bleeding by simply omitting gluten and sugar from their diets.

Gluten is found in wheat, barley, oats, rye, kamut and spelt. It can be found in "hidden" sources such as hydrolyzed vegetable protein, textured vegetable protein and hydrolyzed plant protein. Some forms of malt, modified food starch, soy sauces, grain vinegar, binders, fillers and "natural" flavorings can also have a gluten base. Be sure to read all labels. Appendix A gives recommendations for gluten-free products that actually taste good.

Several organizations are available to help people deal with gluten intolerances. The Celiac Sprue Foundation in Studio City, California is an excellent resource. Please see Appendix E for more information.

MAINTENANCE PLAN
IMMUNE SUPPORT
I recommend the use of glyconutrients, garlic and a whole foods diet to support the immune system.

EFAS
I recommend the use of flaxseed oil on a daily basis. Some women also benefit from Evening of Primrose oil. In my testing the fish oils rarely test as well as the flaxseed oil. Fish swim in polluted water. The fish oil comes from the liver, which is also a detox organ in fish. Consequently the chance of containing toxins is higher in fish oil than in organic flaxseed oil.

EFAs help to decrease sugar cravings and support the skin.

PROTEIN POWDER
Added protein powder can help support the body, especially if it is in a predigested form or from a vegetable base. I usually add this

to a smoothie. If a person has trouble digesting the protein powder, they may need to work with an amino acid supplement.

PROBIOTICS
Probiotic support is crucial to maintain the good flora in the bowel, especially if enemas and/or colonics are done. Most people benefit from ongoing probiotic support. Probiotics are destroyed by excessive stress, antibiotics, birth control pills, many medications, carbonated beverages (i.e., soda) and sugar.

DIGESTIVE ENZYMES
If there is any trouble with digestion after a cleanse, add a digestive enzyme. Undigested food sets the stage for an increase in toxic load and allergic reactions.

FIBER
Even if a high fiber diet is followed, many people benefit from supplemental fiber. Fiber must always be taken thirty minutes before taking supplements or medications. Fibers should be varied. Be sure to consume adequate water to prevent any bloating.

EXERCISE
The higher levels of oxygen from exercise discourages the growth of any unhealthy "critter" in the body. Exercise can be as simple as walking. The key is regularity.

NOTES FOR CHAPTER SIX

1. Lono Kahuna Kupua A'o, *Don't Drink the Water* (Pagos Springs, CO: Kali Press, 1998), p. 43.

2. Bruce Fife, N.D., *The Detox Book: How to Detoxify Your Body to Improve Your Health, Stop Disease, and Reverse Aging* (Colorado Springs, CO: HealthWise Publications, 1997), p. 94.

3. Ibid., p. 178.

RECOMMENDATIONS & RESOURCES

APPENDIX A
RECOMMENDED PRODUCTS
✦✦✦

SUPPLEMENTS

CANDIDA CLEANSE
YeastMAX
YeastMAX by Advanced Naturals is our favorite cleanse. It has been formulated by Brenda Watson, C.T. (colon therapist) and Leonard Smith, M.D. Brenda Watson is President of the International Association of Colon Therapy and founder of five natural health clinics specializing in internal cleansing and detoxification. Dr. Smith is a gastrointestinal surgeon and serves as Medical Advisor for Advanced Naturals.

YST/CAN and LVR/DRN
YST/CAN and LVR/DRN are homeopathic cleanse supports from Apex. The YST/CAN works as the cleanse and LVR/DRN works as the liver drainage support. The combination of the two works well with blood type O's or where chemical/mercury toxicity is contributing to the fungal growth.

GLYCONUTRIENTS
Ambrotose
Ambrotose (contains eight essential saccharides — a glyconutrient

---

product) by Mannatech is available from local associates or from Lifestyle for Health.

Several products on the market contain one of the eight essential saccharides. The single saccharide found in many of these products is mannose. I have found it far superior to use all eight of the essential saccharides. My recommendation for this support is Ambrotose by Mannatech, a product which contains all eight essential saccharides and holds the composition patent for these saccharides.

IMMUNE BUILDERS
Kyolic Aged Garlic
Kyolic Aged Garlic is available from local health food stores.

Barlean's Green
Barlean's Green (an excellent green powder) is available from local health food stores and from Lifestyle for Health.

KyoGreen
KyoGreen (an excellent green powder) is available from local health food stores and from Lifestyle for Health.

EFAS
Barlean's Flaxseed Oil
Barlean's High Lignan Flaxseed oil is widely available from local health food stores and from Lifestyle for Health.

PROTEIN
Naturade Protein Powder
Naturade Protein Powder is a vegetable-based protein powder. It is available in local health food stores and from Lifestyle for Health.

PROBIOTICS
FloraMAX
FloraMAX is a natural probiotic by Advanced Naturals. It contains five strains of digestive flora which are native to the human digestive tract. It also includes F.O.S. to support growth of healthy bac-

teria. L-glutamine and N-acetyl-glucosamine are included to assist the body in maintaining a healthy digestive tract.

Kyodophilus
Kyodophilus (a probiotic that does not require refrigeration) is widely available in local health food stores and from Lifestyle for Health.

Megadophilus and Bifido
Natren Megadophilus (small intestine support) and Bifido (large intestine support) is available in local health food stores and from Lifestyle for Health.

MINERALS
Trace Minerals
ConcenTrace Trace Minerals mineral drops are available in local health food stores and from Lifestyle for Health.

ENZYMES
Enzyme Solutions
Enzyme Solutions by 21st Century has a full line of enzymes. We use this line exclusively for enzyme support. The questionnaire and testing methods taught by Dr. Loomis provide the basis to determine which enzyme to use. For carbohydrate digestion Enzyme Solution #14 is used. For fat and protein digestion Enzyme Solution #11 is used. For addressing reflux, either Enzyme Solution #12 (if there is a history of antacid use) or #32 (if there is no history of antacids) is used.

FIBER
FiberMAX
FiberMAX by Advanced Naturals is a unique, dietary fiber made from flax seeds. It also contains acidophilus and bifidus (probiotic support) and amino acids to support a healthy digestive lining. It is available in powder or capsule form.

PARASITE CLEANSES
ParaMAX
ParaMAX by Advanced Naturals is a natural parasite cleanse to support a healthy balance of intestinal flora and organisms. No fasting is necessary with this product; however, following the Candida diet is helpful.

ParaGONE
ParaGONE for Kids by Advanced Naturals is formulated for children ages 4 to 12. This two-part formula has a tasty cherry-flavored liquid and tiny, easy-to-swallow capsules.

Nature's Sunshine
Nature's Sunshine carries each of the recommend herbs for parasite cleansing: black walnut, wormwood and cloves.

ENDOCRINE SUPPORT
Plus
Plus (contains glyconutrients) by Mannatech is available from associates and from Lifestyle for Health.

Sport
Sport by Mannatech (contains glyconutrients) is available from associates and from Lifestyle for Health.

LYMPH SUPPORT
Mucouslysis
Mucouslysis (concentrated mucous dissolver homeopathic) by Genex is available from Lifestyle for Health.

Lympho Liquitrophic
Lympho Liquitrophic (lymph drainage homeopathic) by Genex is available from Lifestyle for Health.

LFH COACHING
LFH Coaches are trained to work with people both in the office and long distance. If you would like help in identifying the best cleanse and support protocol for you, call the LFH office. Check out the LFH website for information on LFH Coaches around the country.

FOOD MANUFACTURERS
Alta Dena
Alta Dena has a great line of quality dairy products, from fresh milk to kefir, yogurt, ice cream and others. They are committed to producing quality milk products without using bovine growth hormones. Dairy products produced without this hormone are much safer for you and your family. Alta Dena's quality and integrity are excellent.

Alta Dena Certified Dairy
17637 Valley Boulevard
City of Industry, CA 91744-5731
Voice: 800-533-2479
Web: www.altadenadairy.com

Barbara's Bakery
Barbara's Bakery provides quality, nutritious foods, from chips, pretzels and cookies to cereals, granola bars, bread sticks and crackers. Their food is tasty and very reasonably priced. Many low-fat and no-fat foods are available.

Barbara's Bakery, Inc.
3900 Cypress Drive
Petaluma, CA 94954
Voice: 707-765-2273

Cascadian Farm
Cascadian Farm provides a wealth of excellent products. Many of their products are organic, from their frozen fruits and vegetables to their jams, jellies, preserves, sorbets, pickles and relishes. They

have great "popsicles" made with organic milk and unrefined sugar. They have Kosher foods.

Cascadian Farm
P.O. Box 568
Concrete, WA 98237
Voice: 800-869-7105
Web: www.cfarm.com

Coleman Natural Meats
Coleman Natural Meats come from totally natural cattle, raised without hormones or steroids. The flavor is excellent, beyond comparison with other meats. They provide beef and other meats.

Coleman Natural Meats Inc.
5140 Race Court #4
Denver, CO 80127
Voice: 303-297-9393
Fax: 303-297-0426
Web: www.colemannatural.com

Frontier Herbs
Frontier provides fresh herbs in both bulk and packaged forms. They also produce organic coffees. This company is committed to quality and integrity.

Frontier Cooperatives Herbs
1 Frontier Road
P.O. Box 299
Norway, IA 52318
Voice: 800-729-5422

Horizon
Horizon is a supplier of all-organic dairy products. They are cow, not goat, based and include a full line of milk, cheese and yogurt.

Horizon
Boulder, CO 80301
Voice: 800-237-2711
Web: www.horizonorganic.com

Mori Nu

Mori Nu has the best silken tofu (a smooth tofu that has the texture of sour cream, without the cholesterol). Mori Nu tofu works the best with many of my recipes. It comes in aseptic packaging for longer shelf life. Their "lite" tofu has the least fat of any tofu on the market.

Mori Nu
2050 West 190th, #110
Torrance, CA 90504
Voice: 800-669-8638
Fax: 310-787-2727

Mountain Sun

Mountain Sun is committed to producing organic products. They provide great organic and natural food juices under the labels of Mountain Sun and Apple Hill. Their flavors and their varieties are superb.

Mountain Sun
18390 Highway 145
Dolores, CO 81323
Voice: 303-882-2283
Web: www.morinu.com

Muir Glen

Muir Glen tomato products are by far my favorite. These organically grown tomato products are packaged in enamel lined cans, a detail which produces a superior taste and product. Muir Glen products range from chunky tomato sauces to tomato paste to whole tomatoes. Throw away those tinny-tasting tomatoes today and try Muir Glen.

Muir Glen
424 North 7th Street
Sacramento, CA 95814
Voice: 800-832-6345
Fax: 916-557-0903
Web: www.muirglen.com

Pamela's Products

Pamela's Products produces our favorite cookies. Many of their cookies are wheat-free, sugar-free and some are dairy-free. A line of biscotti cookies has been added to the regular line.

Pamela's Products
335 Allerton Avenue
South San Francisco, CA 94080
Voice: 650-952-4546
Web: www.pamelasproducts.com

Pasta Riso

Pasta Riso is the only brown rice pasta I've tasted that tastes good. This line of pastas comes in all of the basic shapes as well as an organic 5-vegetable shell. Be sure to follow their recommended cooking directions.

Pasta Riso
Rice Inventions Inc.
Pickering Postal Station
P.O. Box 16
Pickering, Ontario
Canada L1V 2R2

San-J

San-J has great sauces for stir-fries and marinades. Their tamari has an excellent flavor and will quickly replace your sodium-laden soy sauces. Their Thai peanut sauce is great for stir-fries and excellent in salads. Their miso soup is a delicious cup-a-soup.

San-J International, Inc.
2880 Sprouse Drive
Richmond, VA 23231
Voice: 800-446-5500
Web: www.san-j.com

Shelton

Shelton poultry products are raised without antibiotics and are free-range grown. They are raised without hormones, or growth stimulants — which are common in most other commercially raised chickens and turkeys. ("All Natural" on a poultry label is defined by the Department of Agriculture as "minimally processed with no artificial ingredients." This claim on a whole bird only means that the bird has not been artificially basted, which is basically meaningless.) Shelton provides fresh poultry and other poultry-related products. Their chicken broth is excellent.

Shelton Poultry
204 Loranne
Pomona, CA 91767
Voice: 800-541-1833
Web: www.sheltons.com

Spectrum Naturals
Spectrum Naturals' oils are expeller pressed without solvents. Both refined and unrefined oils are available. Their products range from oils and supplemental oils to cheese, mayonnaise, vinegars, dressings and sauces. Their brand names include Spectrum Naturals (oils), Veg-Omega, Sonnet Farms (cheese), Ayla's Organic (dressings) and Blue Banner.

Spectrum Naturals, Inc.
133 Copeland Street
Petaluma, CA 94952
Voice: 800-995-2705
Fax: 707-765-1026
Web: www.spectrumnaturals.com

Sunspire
Sunspire is your answer to sugar-laden chocolate. Sunspire products contain no refined sugar and taste great. They can be purchased in carob, chocolate, mint and peanut. They provide confections and chocolate chips. They have many dairy-free products.

Sunspire
2114 Adams Avenue
San Leandro, CA 94577
Voice: 510-569-9731

VitaSpelt

VitaSpelt produces some of the best whole-grain pastas. They use whole-grain spelt, which many wheat-sensitive people can tolerate. Be sure to not overcook whole-grain pasta, as that will make it mushy. They have added a new focacia bread, which can be used as an excellent pizza base. I have prepared many recipes for Vita-Spelt products.

VitaSpelt
Purity Foods Inc.
2871 West Jolly Road
Okemos, Ml 48864
Voice: 800-99-SPELT

Westbrae and Little Bear

Westbrae and Little Bear are excellent brands. The company is committed to organic and low-fat products. Little Bear, under the brand Bearitos, has excellent chips, taco shells, tostada shells, popcorn, salsa, refried beans and pretzels. They also produce a licorice without refined sugar and additives. Westbrae has excellent snack food, cookies, soy milk, soy beverages and condiments.

Little Bear/Westbrae
1065 East Walnut Street
Carson, CA 90746
Voice: 800-776-1276
Web: www.westbrae.com

APPENDIX B
CLEANSING EQUIPMENT
✦✦✦

The following equipment has been mentioned throughout this book as being helpful to those in the process of cleansing. This resource list is not meant to be exhaustive of all possible sources, however, I do recommend these particular sources.

AIR FILTERS

The portable air filter we use was purchased from Sears, provides negative ions and was under $100.00. Other quality air filters can be purchased from:

> **Alpine Air Purifiers**
> Frankly Healthy
> Aurora, CO 80012
> Voice: 303-696-2082

> **Allergy Free**
> 1502 Pine Drive
> Dickinson, TX 77539
> Voice: 800-ALLERGY

To further cleanse the environment, I recommend a zeolite rock sold by Natural NonScents. It is effective at removing chemicals, electro magnetic fields and odors.

Natural NonScents
Voice: 303-794-4477

COLEMA BOARDS

Jubilee Co-op
10244 South Progress Lane
Parker, CO 80134
Voice: 303-805-1618

ENEMA BAGS

The Fleet enema bag is good for enemas and can be easily found in drug stores, such as Walgreens, Payless and in some grocery stores.

HOUSEHOLD CLEANERS

Many excellent companies provide toxin-free household cleaners. These companies include Shaklee, Amway and Ecover.

LAUNDRY PRODUCTS

Many excellent companies provide non-toxic laundry products. These include Shaklee, Amway and Ecover. I never recommend using dryer sheets, as they can aggravate skin problems due to the perfumes and chemicals.

LIVER PACKS

Caster oil can be used for liver packs. Caster oil can be purchased in pharmacies and health food or grocery stores. The best source for organic, expeller pressed caster oil is the Heritage Store.

Heritage Store
Voice: 800-862-2923

REBOUNDER

Rebounders can be found in discount stores, such as Walmart, and sporting good stores. These are not effective and can actually damage the spine. Professional quality rebounders are essential for safety and maximum health benefits. They are available from Lifestyle for Health.

LFH
6520 South Broadway
Littleton, CO 80121
Voice: 303-794-4477

SHOWER HEADS & BATH BALLS

There are many shower heads on the market today. A good brand is New Wave, which can be found in health food stores or purchased from Lifestyle from Health.

If a person is doing detox baths, the water should be purified. If a whole house system is not available, I recommend New Wave bath balls. They can be purchased from Lifestyle for Health.

WATER FILTERS

We have chosen a three-stage, reverse osmosis water filtration system from Shaklee called BestWater. To find the most recent ratings, check the most current issue of *Consumer Report* magazine covering this topic.

For bottled water I recommend Trinity which can be found in all health food stores and some grocery stores.

Appendix C
Candida Recipes
♦♦♦

For a complete set of recipes, I recommend getting a copy of my *Lifestyle for Health Cookbook.* It can be found in health food stores or by calling Lifestyle for Health. Here is a collection of favorite recipes.

Breakfast
Breakfast Suggestions
- ♦ Smoothie
- ♦ Hot Cereal (oatmeal, kamut, whole grains)
- ♦ Eggs

Breakfast Recipes
Candida Cleanse Fruit Smoothie
1 – 1½ c. liquid (water, almond milk, rice milk, soy milk *or* fruit juice)
½ banana (optional)
¼ – ½ c. fresh or frozen fruit
ice
Cell Essentials™
optional additions

1. Blend in blender.

Cell Essentials™ for Smoothies
1 – 2 scoops of protein powder
1 – 2 Tbl. of flaxseed oil (recommend Barlean's Flaxseed oil)
¼ – ½ tsp. of glyconutrients (recommend Ambrotose™ by Mannatech)

Optional Ingredients for Smoothies
10 – 20 drops of Trace Minerals ConcenTrace Drops
1 – 3 tsp. of a green powder
1 tsp. colostrum

Notes
- ♦ Change the liquid source and the fruits you use for variety and flavor.
- ♦ Learn to make a smoothie in such a way that you enjoy it. It can be delicious and great for you!
- ♦ During travel, the basic smoothie can be placed in a shaker and shaken.

Makes 1 smoothie for an adult.
Makes enough for 2 children.

Kamut Cereal
1 c. water
sprinkle of salt
⅓ c. Bob's Red Mill Kamut Farina

1. Add salt to water and bring water to a boil.
2. Add kamut cereal.
3. Lower heat and simmer, partially covered, for 8 to 9 minutes. Stir occasionally.
4. Sweeten cereal with stevia to taste and add soy or rice milk as desired.

Serves 1.

Baked Apple Pancake

2 Tbl. clarified butter†
4 large eggs
½ c. brown rice *or* barley flour
¼ tsp. sea salt
½ c. soy milk *or* rice milk
1 tsp. vanilla
5 – 20 drops of stevia, optional
½ Granny Smith apple, thinly sliced

1. Preheat oven to 450°.
2. Place clarified butter in an 8" pan and place in oven to get hot.
3. Beat eggs until light, add all ingredients except apples and beat on high for 2 minutes.
4. Place apples in pan, pour batter over top.
5. Bake 18 to 20 minutes or until golden brown.
6. For Candida diet, squeeze fresh lemon juice on top of pancake. For non-Candida diet, top with applesauce and sprinkle with cinnamon.

† To make clarified butter, melt butter and remove the milk solids that form at the top.

Serves 4.

Granola-like Breakfast

4 Tbl. sesame seeds
4 Tbl. sunflower seeds
4 Tbl. flaxseeds
4 c. rolled oats
¼ c. soy milk
cinnamon to taste

1. Grind seeds in seed grinder or clean coffee grinder.

2. Combine ground seeds with rolled oats and divide into 2 equal portions.
3. Soak one portion in soy milk.
4. Place both portions in refrigerator overnight.
5. To serve, stir portions together, sweeten with stevia, top with plain yogurt.

Note
- ♦ Adapted from *Flax for Life* by Jade Beutler.

Serves 3 – 4.

Easy Veggie and Egg Frittata

¼ c. chopped red onion
½ c. chopped green *or* red pepper
oil or water
1 c. chopped tomatoes
8 eggs
¼ c. plain yogurt, goat yogurt *or* soy yogurt, if tolerated
1 tsp. Italian herbs
1 c. grated soy cheese *or* rice mozzarella cheese

1. Sauté onion and pepper in oil or water.
2. Stir in tomatoes and remove from heat. Place half in lightly oiled oven casserole dish.
3. Mix eggs, yogurt and herbs in blender and pour mixture over tomatoes.
4. Mix remaining half of tomatoes and cheese and pour over top of frittata.
5. Bake at 350° for 15 to 20 minutes.

Note
- ♦ An easy, delicious breakfast choice.

Serves 4 – 6.

Asparagus Strata
    1 Tbl. butter *or* oil, optional
    ½ c. water
    5 c. sliced asparagus (1½ pounds)
    2 c. leeks, sliced (3 small)
    3 Tbl. chopped parsley
    ½ tsp. dried tarragon
    1 tsp. grated lemon rind
    ¼ tsp. salt
    pepper, optional
    12 oz. *thin* slices yeast-free bread (i.e., French Meadow)
    1 c. soy cheese
    2½ c. soy milk *or* rice milk
    3 eggs
    1 egg white
    1½ c. fresh breadcrumbs (about 3 slices) from yeast-free bread

1. Sauté asparagus and leeks in butter and water. Simmer about 10 minutes or until done.
2. Stir in parsley, tarragon, lemon, salt, pepper
3. Arrange half of bread slices in single layer in lightly oiled 13" x 9" pan.
4. Top with half of asparagus mixture and ½ cup of the cheese. Repeat.
5. Combine milk, eggs and egg white and mix. Pour mixture over strata.
6. Cover, chill for 8 hours.
7. Sprinkle with bread crumbs.
8. Bake at 400°, uncovered for 40 minutes.

Note
   ♦ This is a good company dish.

Serves 6.

LUNCH
LUNCH IDEAS
Dips
- Be creative with veggie dips.
- Dilute dips into salad dressings with broth or veggie juices.

Salads
- Add cooked chicken, turkey or grilled salmon to salads.
- Nuts, cooked whole grains or cooked eggs can be added to vegetarian salads for additional protein.
- Try using three to five kinds of greens in salads (i.e., butter, green or red leaf, Romaine, spinach, chard, kale, escarole, mixed greens, cabbage, red or Nappa cabbage).

Soups
- Add leftover grains, veggies or beans to veggie or chicken broth for a quick soup. If leftovers cause a digestion problem, make the soup after a dinner, freeze and use later.

Sandwiches
- Instead of yeast bread, use spelt tortillas for the base.
- Instead of mayonnaise, use humus for a basic spread.
- Make quick burritos by wrapping cooked, mashed beans with grated veggies in tortillas.
- Use tortillas as a pizza base, top with pizza sauce (check ingredients), grated veggies and broil.

LUNCH RECIPES
Homemade Salsa
3 tomatoes, diced
4 sprigs cilantro *or* parsley
½ medium onion, diced
1 green onion, chopped
1 small jalapeno pepper, chopped
½ c. Muir Glen tomato sauce

3 Tbl. Barlean's flaxseed oil

1. Combine tomatoes, cilantro, onion, scallion and jalapeno in blender or food processor and process until chunky.
2. In separate bowl, mix tomato sauce and flax oil.
3. Mix both mixtures together. Chill.

Note
   ♦ Adapted from *Flax for Life* by Jade Beutler.

Makes 2 cups.

Guacamole Dip
   1 mashed avocado
   ½ tsp. Mexican seasoning
   ½ tsp. cumin
   ½ tsp. dried oregano
   1 Tbl. Barlean's flaxseed oil

1. Mix all together and serve with raw veggies.

Makes about ¾ cup.

Avocado Dressing
   1 avocado
   1 clove garlic, minced
   2 Tbl. oil
   2 tsp. fresh lemon juice
   1 tsp. dill weed
   sea salt to taste

1. Blend all in food processor. Add water to thin.

Makes about ¾ cup.

Yummy Green Dip

2 c. packed spinach leaves
¾ c. packed parsley
3 Tbl. lemon juice
1 tsp. basil
½ tsp. cumin
1 clove garlic, minced
½ c. olive oil

1. Blend all in blender until smooth.
2. Serve as dip or dressing.

Makes about 2 cups.

Humus

1 c. cooked garbanzo beans, drained
½ c. tahini (sesame seed paste)
¼ c. bean juice *or* water
2 – 3 Tbl. fresh lemon juice
1 – 2 Tbl. olive oil
2 – 4 cloves garlic
½ tsp. sea salt to taste
cayenne pepper to taste

1. Blend all in blender. If too stiff, add a little more water or bean water.
2. Refrigerate several hours.

Note
♦ Freezes well.

Variations
♦ 1 to 2 Tbl. flaxseed oil can be added to basic recipe.
♦ For a Pesto-type Humus, add:
   1 c. lightly packed fresh basil leaves

1 c. lightly packed fresh parsley leaves
Steam basil and parsley leaves for 10 seconds. Drain and
add to humus mixture.

♦ For a Pasta Sauce:
Reserve additional ½ c. bean juice.
Add juice to Pesto-type Humus blend.
Add 1 c. water, 1 Tbl. olive oil and stir into cooked pasta.

Makes 2 cups.

Black Bean and Corn Salad

1 c. water
¼ tsp. cumin seeds
½ c. quinoa
1 c. black beans, cooked
1 c. corn
1 red pepper, chopped
1 tomato, chopped
2 Tbl. red onion, minced
½ tsp. sea salt
2 Tbl. white sesame seeds
1 Tbl. lemon juice
2 Tbl. olive oil
2 – 4 c. fresh greens

1. Bring water to boil. Add cumin and quinoa.
2. Lower heat and simmer for 20 minutes. Fluff cooked mixture
   with fork, cool.
3. Rinse beans and combine with corn, pepper, tomato, onion and
   quinoa.
4. Mix salt, seeds, lemon juice and olive oil.
5. Toss salad dressing with the bean mixture. Serve on a bed of
   greens.

Serves 4.

Fiesta Salad

6 c. mixed greens
1½ c. tomatoes, chopped
⅔ c. corn
½ c. yellow pepper, julienned
½ c. red pepper, julienned
1 bunch green onions, sliced
⅓ c. salsa made without vinegar (or a vinegar-free dressing)
⅓ c. plain or soy yogurt

1. Combine veggies.
2. Mix salsa and yogurt and drizzle over veggies.
3. Serve with corn chips.

Serves 4.

Easy Vegetable Soup

1 onion, sautéed in oil
3 medium sweet potatoes, peeled and chopped
3 zucchini, chopped
1 – 2 c. chopped broccoli
3 cans chicken broth
2 medium potatoes, peeled and shredded
½ tsp. celery seed
2 tsp. salt
1 tsp. cumin
pepper, optional
1 c. milk

1. Sauté onion in small amount of oil or water.
2. Place onion and all other veggies in crock pot.
3. Pour broth and spices over and mix well.
4. Cover and cook on low 8 to 10 hours, 4 to 5 hours on high.
5. Add milk and cook 30 to 60 minutes.

Note

◆ If too thin, mix 1 Tbl. arrowroot powder or cornstarch into a small amount of water until blended. Stir into soup and simmer until thickened.

Serves 6.

Quick Chili

1 pound ground turkey *or* 2 c. TVP (follow manufacturer's directions)
1 onion, chopped
3 – 4 cans chili beans
1 28 oz. can Muir Glen ground tomatoes
1 Tbl. chili powder
1 tsp. ground cumin
1 tsp. salt, optional, to taste

1. Sauté onion and ground turkey together.
2. Add chili beans, tomatoes and seasonings. Mix well.
3. Place into crock pot.
4. Cover and cook for 6 to 8 hours on low or for 3 to 4 hours on high.

Serves 4 – 6.

Easy Spinach and Chicken Soup

6 c. chicken broth
1 c. water
1 c. sliced green onions
1 c. brown rice pasta
6 c. spinach, coarsely cut
2 skinless, boneless chicken breasts (about 12 ounces), sliced into julienne strips
1 tomato, seeded and diced

1. Bring stock, water and green onions to boil.
2. Add pasta and cook according to directions.
3. Add spinach and boil for 1 minute.
4. Add chicken and bring to boil.
5. Cover, set off of heat and let steam for 5 minutes.
6. Stir in tomatoes.
7. Season to taste and serve.

Serves 6.

Turkey Stew
8 oz. dry white navy beans
4 c. chicken broth
2 carrots, cut into 1" pieces
1 stalk celery, thinly sliced
1 medium onion, chopped
¼ tsp. dried thyme
2 bay leaves
3 whole cloves
1½ pounds turkey breast, cut in small ½" slices
1 small tomato, seeded and chopped
¼ c. fresh parley leaves, chopped
2 cloves garlic, minced

1. Place washed beans in pot with broth, carrots, celery, onion, thyme, bay leaves and whole cloves.
2. Bring mixture to a boil, reduce heat and simmer for 90 minutes (this can be done in a crock pot). Stir 2 or 3 times during cooking time.
3. Add turkey, tomato, parsley and garlic. Boil for 5 to 7 minutes or until turkey is done.
4. Remove bay leaves, whole cloves and serve.

Serves 4 – 6.

Spelt Tortillas
   2 c. spelt flour
   ¾ c. hot water
   1½ tsp. baking powder
   3 Tbl. oil
   1 tsp. salt

Bosch Method
1. In large Bosch, make three to six times the recipe (increase ingredient amounts to make three to six times, as you prefer).
2. Add hot water and all remaining ingredients but spelt flour in order listed.
3. Add enough spelt flour to make a *very* sticky dough. Dough must be very sticky.
4. Put into an oiled baggie and let rest 20 minutes.
5. Cut into balls about the size of kiwi, flatten and cook on both sides.

Manual Method
1. Place flour, baking powder and salt in bowl.
2. Mix in oil by hand and mix until well blended.
3. Add hot water until a sticky dough forms. Dough must be very sticky.
4. Put into an oiled baggie and let rest 20 minutes.
5. Cut into balls about the size of kiwi, flatten and cook on both sides.

Notes
   ♦ I recommend the Tortilla Chef to flatten and cook tortillas quickly — for more information on the Tortilla Chef, contact the Lifestyle for Health office.
   ♦ These are a great alternative to wheat-based tortillas.
   ♦ These freeze well.

Each recipe makes 8 – 12 tortillas.

DINNER
DINNER IDEAS
- Grill chicken, turkey or fish and add a vegetable and salad.
- Stir fry favorite veggies and serve over whole grains.
- Make tacos using cooked quinoa (use 1 part quinoa to 2 parts water, bring to boil, cover, simmer for 20 minutes), lettuce, soft taco shells, chopped tomato and soy cheese.
- Use vegetarian patties in sandwiches, added to soups or as a main entree.

DINNER RECIPES
Onion Sauce
2 Tbl. olive oil
1 medium onion, thin slices
¼ tsp. thyme
1 c. chicken broth *or* veggie broth
2 Tbl. Barlean's flaxseed oil

1. Sauté onion in oil until lightly caramelized. Stir in thyme.
2. Add stock, bring to a boil and simmer for 3 to 4 minutes.
3. Puree in blender, adding flaxseed oil at end.

Note
- This is great on veggies or for dipping artichokes.

Makes 1½ cups.

Ratatouille
1 whole eggplant, chopped
1 red pepper, chopped
1 green pepper, chopped
4 medium tomatoes, seeded, cut into wedges
1 medium yellow squash, thick slices
2 medium zucchini, thick slices

2 onions, chopped
1 – 2 Tbl. olive oil
1 whole bay leaf
1 tsp. basil
1 tsp. parsley
¼ tsp. oregano

1. Mix all veggies together in bowl.
2. Sprinkle oil and herbs onto veggies and stir to mix.
3. Place in lightly oiled baking dish.
4. Bake at 375° for 30 to 60 minutes or until veggies are as tender as desired. Stir occasionally.
5. Serve hot or cold.

Variations
- ♦ Place on spelt tortillas and bake as a pizza.
- ♦ Place on broiled polenta topped with a pasta sauce.
- ♦ Leftovers can be added to soups.

Serves 4 – 6.

Chili Rellenos Casserole
1 can vegetarian refried beans
1 4 oz. can mild green chilies, chopped
5 oz. soy *or* rice cheese
1½ c. cooked brown rice, quinoa *or* a combination of the two grains
2 c. enchilada sauce (or tomato sauce seasoned with Mexican seasoning)

1. Layer the refried beans in the bottom of a 9" square pan (lightly oiled).
2. Top with chilies, cheese, grains and sauce.
3. Bake at 350° for 25 to 30 minutes.

Note
- ♦ This recipe freezes well. It can be doubled and frozen before baking.

Variations
- ♦ Cooked ground turkey can be layered into filling for a non-vegetarian variation.
- ♦ Serve topped with chopped lettuce, chopped tomato and corn chips for a quick meal.

Serves 4 – 6.

Oat Nut Patties
1½ c. pecan pieces *or* walnut pieces
2 c. oats
3 eggs *or* egg substitute
½ c. soy milk *or* rice milk
½ c. chopped onion
3 green onions, thin slices
1 tsp. sage
1 tsp. sea salt, to taste

1. Combine all ingredients.
2. Chill a couple of hours or overnight.
3. Form into patties and brown in skillet.

Variation
- ♦ Simmer browned patties in chicken or vegetable stock for about 20 minutes.

Makes 6 – 8 patties.

Oven Baked Chicken

1¼ c. ground corn flakes *or* other grain, ground in blender
¼ c. spelt flour
1½ Tbl. parsley
1 tsp. paprika
¾ tsp. oregano
¾ tsp. basil
½ tsp. sea salt
chicken pieces

1. Mix first seven ingredients in baggie.
2. Toss chicken pieces into bag and mix.
3. Place on lightly oiled pan.
4. Bake at 350° for 30 minutes, turn chicken over and bake until done, about 30 minutes.

Variation

♦ Mix ½ to 1 package taco mix with ground corn flakes. Proceed according to above directions.

Makes 1½ cups mix.

Baked Fish

1 pound firm flesh fish (salmon, tuna, halibut)
2 medium zucchini, grated
1 Tbl. parsley
2 green onions, sliced

1. Place fish in lightly oiled, shallow baking pan.
2. Mix together the zucchini, parsley and onion. Place on top of the fish.
3. Bake at 400° for 15 minutes.

Serves 4.

Red Beans and Rice

2 c. red beans
6 c. water
1 onion, chopped
1 stalk celery, thin slices
2 cloves garlic, minced
¼ c. red pepper, minced
¼ c. chopped tomatoes
1 tsp. Mexican seasoning

1. Cook beans in crock pot or soup pot until tender.
2. Sauté onion, celery and garlic in oil or water until tender. Add peppers and sauté until tender.
3. Mix veggies, tomatoes, seasoning and beans in pot (or crock-pot) and cook on low for 4 to 6 hours.
4. Serve over hot rice, millet or quinoa. Cayenne pepper can be added for extra hotness.

Serves 4 – 6.

Stuffed Peppers

2 whole peppers
¾ pound ground turkey, optional
1 leek, cleaned and sliced thin
2 cloves garlic, minced
½ c. tomatoes, seeded, chopped
1½ c. cooked rice *or* quinoa
1 Tbl. basil
1 Tbl. parsley
1 8 oz. can tomato sauce
¼ c. chopped fresh parley

1. Halve peppers and steam until tender crisp.
2. Brown turkey, leek and garlic. Add tomatoes and spices.
3. Stir in cooked grain and fill peppers.

4. Place peppers in oven dish, pour tomato sauce around. Sprinkle with fresh parsley.
5. Bake at 350° for 15 to 30 minutes.

Serves 3.

MORE IDEAS

For other recipe ideas, be sure to check out *Lifestyle for Health Cookbook, Meals in 30 Minutes, Kid Smart!,* by Cheryl Townsley, and *Flax for Life* by Jade Beutler. All books can be found in local health food stores or by calling Lifestyle for Health.

SURPRISE ... TREATS!
Yummy, Legal Cake
   1½ c. barley flour *or* brown rice flour
   2 Tbl. arrowroot powder
   1 Tbl. baking powder
   6 eggs, separated
   ½ c. oil *or* clarified butter†
   ⅓ c. fresh lemon juice
   1 Tbl. vanilla
   5 Tbl. vegetable glycerine‡
   10 – 20 drops of stevia, optional

1. Mix dry ingredients in bowl.
2. Beat egg whites until stiff.
3. Beat egg yolk until thick, add oil, juice, vanilla, glycerine and stevia to yolks and mix well.
4. Add yolk mixture to dry ingredients and blend well.
5. Fold flour mixture into egg whites.
6. Pour batter into oiled angel food cake pan or 9" round pan.
7. Bake at 350° for 35 minutes or until done.
8. Cool for ten minutes and remove from pan.

† Clarified butter can be made by melting butter and removing the foam (milk solids). Once clarified, it can be stored in the fridge.

‡ Vegetable glycerine is a vegetable oil derived from coconut oil that helps stabilize baked goods. It is also a sweetener — one tablespoon of vegetable glycerine is equivalent to four tablespoons of sugar. It can usually be found in the specialty isle or health and beauty isle of most health food stores. Common brands are Heritage, NOW or Starwest Botanicals.

Note

♦ For more sweetness, you might want to add a small amount of stevia which is an herb that can add sweetness to a recipe. One teaspoon of stevia is equivalent to one cup of sugar. Stevia is sold as a liquid or as powder and can be found in local health food stores.

Variation

♦ When it is safe to reintroduce some fruit, this cake is delicious when cut in half horizontally and layered with fresh, sliced strawberries.

Serves 8 – 10.

Lemon Frosting

10 Tbl. oil *or* clarified butter†
5 Tbl. vegetable glycerine
1 egg yolk
1½ Tbl. fresh lemon juice

1. Cream oil and glycerine until thick.
2. Beat in egg yolk and lemon juice. Mix well and refrigerate until well chilled.
3. Beat until thick and easy to spread.
4. Frost top of cake and garnish with chopped nuts.

† Clarified butter can be made by melting butter and removing the foam (milk solids). Once clarified, it can be stored in the fridge.

Variation
- ◆ For a sweeter icing, add ½ to 1 tsp. of stevia when mixing the oil and glycerine.

Makes 1⅓ cup.

These desserts were inspired by Gail Burton. For more Candida desserts and other recipes, I highly recommend her book, *The Candida Control Cookbook.*

APPENDIX D
READING & LISTENING MATERIALS
✦✦✦

BOOKS

Anderson, Richard N.D., N.M.D., *Cleanse & Purify Thyself.* 1988.

Baker, Sidney MacDonald, M.D., *Detoxification & Health: The Key to Optimal Health.* New Canaan, CT: Keats Publishing, Inc., 1997.

Braly, James, M.D., *Dr. Braly's Food Allergy & Nutrition Revolution.* New Canaan, CT: Keats Publishing, Inc., 1992.

Burton, Gail, *The Candida Control Cookbook.* Fairfield CT: Aslan Publishing, 1995.

DeCava, Judith A., MS, LNC, *The Real Truth About Vitamins and Antioxidants.* Columbus, GA: Brentwood Academic Press, 1996.

Frähm, David & Anne, *Healthy Habits.* Colorado Springs, CO: Piñon Press, 1993.

Haas, Elson M., M.D., *The Detox Diet.* Berkeley, CA: Celestial Arts, 1996.

Hobbs, Christopher, *Natural Liver Therapy*. Capitola, CA: Botanica Press, 1988.

Jensen, Bernard, DC, *Breathe Again Naturally*. Escondido, CA: Bernard Jensen Enterprises, 1983.

Jerome, Frank J., D.D.S., *Tooth Truth*. San Diego, CA: ProMotion Publishing, 1995.

Kroh, Jacqueline, M.D., *The Whole Way to Natural Detoxification*. Point Roberts, WA: Hartley & Marks Publishers, Inc., 1996.

Moore, Dr. Neecie, *The Facts About Phytochemicals*. Dallas, TX: Charis Publishing Co., 1996.

Morris, Chris, N.D., *The True Nature of Healing*. Menlo Park, CA: The Publications Group, 1997.

Murray, Michael T., N.D. and Jade Beutler, R.R.T., R.C.P., *Understanding Fats & Oils*. Encinitas, CA: Progressive Health Publishing, 1996.

See, Daryl, Ph.D., *For Parents Only*. Lifestyle for Health.

Townsley, Cheryl, N.D., *Discovering Wholeness: The Spirit, Soul and Body Connection*. Littleton, CO: LFH Publishing, 2000.

Townsley, Cheryl, N.D., *Food Puzzle*. Littleton, CO: LFH Publishing, 2001.

Townsley, Cheryl, *Food Smart! Eat Your Way to Better Health*. New York, NY: Tarcher Putnam, 1998.

Townsley, Cheryl, *Kid Smart! Raising a Healthy Child*. Littleton, CO: LFH Publishing, 1996.

Townsley, Cheryl, *Revised Meals in 30 Minutes*. Littleton, CO: LFH Publishing, 1997.

BODY BY DESIGN

If you are ready to invest in all that you can be, allow *Body by Design* to pave the way for you. This do-it-yourself program contains the key principles Cheryl Townsley has distilled from her clinical experience with thousands of clients from around the world. Principles proven to work for real people with real problems.

Body by Design is a complete 10 week program designed to help you "define and recreate you for optimal performance." The program covers, vision and purpose, metabolic profiling, blood type diet basics, Candida and cleansing how-to's, exercise strategies, supplement guidelines, allergy self-testing, and identifying emotional roots to disease, all laid out so that you can customize a program to fit you!

Body by Design can be used by an individual, as a program for a small group to follow, or as an adjunct to our personalized coaching program.

Begin the adventure of designing the rest of your life with Body by Design. Call the Lifestyle for Health office for details and pricing information.

.

CATALOGS

DIAMOND ORGANIC

Diamond Organic provides organic produce by mail.

Diamond Organics
888-ORGANIC

HERITAGE STORE CATALOG

The Heritage Store provides quality, environmentally-safe products including caster oil, ear care, essential oils, homeopathics and much more.

Heritage Store Catalog
800-862-2923

APPENDIX E
HEALTH RESOURCES
& INFORMATION
♦♦♦

NATURAL BIRTH CONTROL RESOURCES

BILLINGS OVULATION METHOD ASSOCIATION
Billings Ovulation Method Association
P.O. Box 16206
St. Paul, MN 55116
Voice: 615-699-8139
Fax: 615-699-8144
Web: boma-usa@quest.net

FERTILITY AWARENESS NETWORK
(National and international resources)
P.O. Box 1190
NY, NY 10009
Voice: 800-597-6267

FERTILITY AWARENESS CENTER
(Seminar information)
P.O. Box 1190
NY, NY 10009
Voice: 212-475-4490
Web: www.fertaware.com

HEALTH-CARE RESOURCES

Lifestyle for Health has compiled a national *Resource Directory* listing health-care providers, co-ops and many products to help on your journey toward health. For more information, or to purchase this directory, call the Lifestyle for Health office at 303-794-4477.

AMERICAN COLLEGE OF NURSE-MIDWIVES

American College of Nurse-Midwives
818 Connecticut Avenue, Suite 900
Washington D.C. 20006
Voice: 202-728-9860
Fax: 202-728-9897
Web: www.midewife.org

AMERICAN OSTEOPATHIC ASSOCIATION

American Osteopathic Association
142 East Ontario Street
Chicago, IL 60611
Voice: 800-621-1773
Web: www.909-net.org

ANOREXIA BULIMIA COUNSELING

Martin Nutritional Counseling
Voice: 314-997-0945

BULIMIA ANOREXIA HELP

St. Johns Behavioral Health
615 South New Ballas Road
Creve Coeur, MO 63141
Voice: 314-569-6565

CELIAC DISEASE FOUNDATION

Celiac Disease Foundation
13251 Ventura Boulevard, Suite 1
Studio City, CA 91604-1838

Voice: 818-990-2354
Fax: 818-990-2379
Email: cdf@celiac.org
Web: www.celiac.org

FEINGOLD ASSOCIATION OF THE U.S.
Feingold Association of the U.S.
P.O. Box 6550
Alexandria, VA 22306
Voice: 703-768-3287
Web: www.feingold.org

INTERNATIONAL COLLEGE OF APPLIED KINESIOLOGY
International College of Applied Kinesiology
6405 Metcalf Avenue, Suite 503
Shawnee Mission, KS 66202-3929
Voice: 913-384-5336
Fax: 913-384-5112
Web: www.icakusa.com

BASTYR UNIVERSITY
Bastyr University
14500 Juanita Drive, NE
Kenmore, WA 98028
Voice: 206-523-9585
Fax: 425-823-6222
Web: www.bastyr.edu

LA LECHE LEAGUE INTERNATIONAL
La Leche League International
1400 North Meacham Road
Schaumburg, IL 60173
Voice: 800-LALECHE
Voice: 847-519-7730
Fax: 847-519-0035
Web: www.lalecheleague.org

USEFUL HEALTH INFORMATION

DETERMINING BLOOD TYPE

    Method 1. Donate blood.

    Method 2. Check with your physician. (They usually do not know. If they run the test, it will cost $200 – $300 and insurance will not cover the charge.)

    Method 3. Purchase a self-test kit from LFH (order form in back of book or via our web site).

APPENDIX F
CANDIDA HISTORY &
CHECKLIST FORMS
♦♦♦

CANDIDA SELF ANALYSIS
The following questionnaire is available on our website at
www.lifestyleforhealth.com.

HISTORY – SECTION 1
This section involves an understanding of your medical history and
how it may have promoted Candida growth. Circle those comment
to which you can answer *yes*. Record your total at the end of the
section.

Points

1. Throughout your lifetime, have you taken any   25
    antibiotics or tetracyclines (Symycin™, Panmycin™,
    Bivramycin™, Monicin™ etc.) for acne or other
    conditions, for more than one month?

2. Have you ever taken a "broad spectrum" antibiotic   20
    for more than two months or four or more times in
    a one-year period? These could include any antibiotics
    taken for respiratory, urinary or other infections.

3. Have you taken a "broad spectrum" antibiotic   6
    — even for a single course? These antibiotics
    include ampicillin™, amoxicillin™, Keflex™, etc.

4. Have you ever had problems with persistent   25
    prostatitis, vaginitis or other problems with
    your reproductive organs?

5. Women — Have you been pregnant:
        Two or more times?   5
        One time?   3

6. Women — Have you taken birth control pills:
        More than two years?   15
        More than six months?   8

7. If you were not breast-fed as an infant.   9

8. Have you taken any cortisone-type drugs   15
    (Prednisone™, Decadron™, etc.)?

9. Are you sensitive to and bothered by exposure
    to perfumes, insecticides or other chemical odors:
        Do you have moderate to severe symptoms?   20
        Do you have mild symptoms?   5

10. Does tobacco smoke bother you?   10

11. Are your symptoms worse on damp, muggy days   20
    or in moldy places?

12. If you have had chronic fungus infections of the
    skin or nails (including athlete's foot, ring worm,
    jock itch), have the infections been:
    Severe or persistent?   20
    Mild to moderate?   10

13. Do you crave sugar (chocolate, ice cream,   10
    candy, cookies, etc.)?

14. Do you crave carbohydrates (bread, bread   10
    and more bread)?

15. Do you crave alcoholic beverages?   10

16. Have you drunk or do you drink chlorinated   20
    water (city or tap)?

Total Score Section 1   _____

Major Symptoms – Section 2

For each of your symptoms, enter the appropriate figure in the point score column.

No symptoms	0
Occasional or mild	3
Frequent and/or moderately severe	6
Severe and/or disabling	9

Points

1. Constipation ____

2. Diarrhea ____

3. Bloating ____

4. Fatigue or lethargy ____

5. Feeling drained ____

6. Poor memory ____

7. Difficulty focusing/brain fog ____

8. Feeling moody or despair ____

9. Numbness, burning or tingling ____

10. Muscle aches ____

11. Nasal congestion or discharge ____

12. Pain and/or swelling in the joints ____

13. Abdominal pain ____

14. Spots in front of the eyes   ____

15. Erratic vision   ____

16. Cold hands and/or feet   ____

Women
17. Endometriosis   ____

18. Menstrual irregularities and/or severe cramps   ____

19. PMS   ____

20. Vaginal discharge   ____

21. Persistent vaginal burning or itching   ____

Men
22. Prostatitis   ____

23. Impotence   ____

Women and Men
24. Loss of sexual desire   ____

25. Low blood sugar   ____

26. Anger or frustration   ____

27. Dry, patchy skin   ____

Total Score Section 2   _____

MINOR SYMPTOMS – SECTION 3

For each of your symptoms, enter the appropriate figure in the point score column.

No symptoms	0
Occasional or mild	1
Frequent and/or moderately severe	2
Severe and/or disabling	3

Points

1. Heartburn   _____

2. Indigestion   _____

3. Belching and intestinal gas   _____

4. Drowsiness   _____

5. Itching   _____

6. Rashes   _____

7. Irritability or jitters   _____

8. Uncoordinated   _____

9. Inability to concentrate   _____

10. Frequent mood swings   _____

11. Postnasal drip   _____

12. Nasal itching   _____

13. Failing vision   _____

14. Burning or tearing of the eyes   _____

15. Recurrent infections of fluid in the ears   _____

16. Ear pain or deafness   _____

17. Headaches   _____

18. Dizziness/loss of balance   _____

19. Pressure above the ears   _____
    (your head feels like it is swelling and tingling)

20. Mucus in the stool   _____

21. Hemorrhoids   _____

22. Dry mouth   _____

23. Rash or blisters in the mouth   _____

24. Bad breath   _____

25. Sore or dry throat   _____

26. Cough   _____

27. Pain or tightness in the chest   _____

28. Wheezing or shortness of breath   _____

29. Urinary urgency or frequency   _____

30. Burning during urination   _____

Total Score Section 3   _____

The Results

Total Score from Section 1	_____
Total Score from Section 2	_____
Total Score from Section 3	_____

Total Score _____

If your score is at least	*Your symptoms are:*
180 Women	Almost certainly yeast connected
140 Men	Almost certainly yeast connected

✦✦✦✦✦✦✦✦✦✦✦✦✦✦✦✦✦✦✦✦✦✦✦✦✦✦✦✦✦✦✦✦✦✦

120 Women	Probably yeast connected
90 Men	Probably yeast connected

✦✦✦✦✦✦✦✦✦✦✦✦✦✦✦✦✦✦✦✦✦✦✦✦✦✦✦✦✦✦✦✦✦✦

60 Women	Possibly yeast connected
40 Men	Possibly yeast connected

✦✦✦✦✦✦✦✦✦✦✦✦✦✦✦✦✦✦✦✦✦✦✦✦✦✦✦✦✦✦✦✦✦✦

If your score is less than	*Your symptoms are:*
60 Women	Probably not yeast connected
40 Men	Probably not yeast connected

If your score is 60+ (women) or 40+ (men), then you will probably want to consider following the suggestions found in this book.

BIBLIOGRAPHY
✦✦✦

Anderson, Dr. Richard N.D., N.M.D., *Cleanse & Purify Thyself.*
1988.

A'o, Lono Kahuna Kupua, *Don't Drink the Water.* Kali Press: Pa-
gosa Springs, CO, 1998.

Baker, Sidney MacDonald, M.D., *Detoxification & Healing: The
Key to Optimal Health.* New Cannaan, CT: Keats Publishing,
Inc., 1997.

Balch, James F., M.D. and Phyllis A. Balch, C.N.C., *Revised and
Expanded Prescription for Nutritional Healing Second Edition.* Garden City, NY: Avery Publishing Group, 1997.

Berkow, Robert M.D., ed. in chief, *The Merck Manual of Medical
Information.* Whitehouse Station, NJ: Merck & CO., Inc.,
1997.

Braly, James, M.D., *Dr. Braly's Food Allergy & Nutrition Revolution.* New Canaan, CT: Keats Publishing, Inc., 1992.

Cassell, Gail, quoted in "Antibiotic Use Must Slow, Experts
Warn," *The Denver Post: August 12, 1998.*

Connolly Pat, *The Candida Albicans Yeast-free Cookbook.* New Canaan, CT: Keats Publishing, Inc., 1985.

Crook, William G. M.D., *Chronic Fatigue Syndrome and the Yeast Connection.* Jackson, TN: Professional Books, 1992.

Crook, William G. M.D., *Yeast Connection.* Jackson, TN: Professional Books, 1986.

D'Adamo, Peter J., N.D., *Eat Right For Your Blood Type.* NY, NY: G.P. Putnam's Sons, 1996.

D'Onofrio, Sal, D.M., D.D., *Yeast Control in Seven Days.* Laguna Beach, CA: (No company), (no date).

Fife, Bruce, N.D., *The Detox Book: How to Detoxify Your Body to Improve Your Health, Stop Disease and Reverse Aging.* Colorado Springs, CO: Healthwise Publications, 1997.

Frähm, David and Anne, *Healthy Habits.* Colorado Springs, CO: Pinon Press, 1993.

Fu, SM and HG Kunkel, "Membrane Immunoglovulin of B Lymphocytes," *J Exp Med*: 1974, 140:894 – 903.

Galland, Leo., M.D., with Dian Dincin Buchman, Ph.D., *Superimmunity for Kids.* NY, NY: Copestone Press, Inc., 1988.

Gittleman, Ann Louise, M.S. with J. Maxwell Desgrey, *Beyond Pritikin.* NY, NY: Bantam Books, 1996.

Gittleman, Ann Louise, M.S., C.N.S., *Get the Sugar Out.* NY, NY: Crown Trade Paperbacks, 1996.

Golan, Ralph, M.D., *Optimal Wellness.* NY, NY: Ballantine Books, 1995.

Haas, Elson, M., M.D., *The Detox Diet.* Berkeley, CA: Celestial Arts, 1996.

Hanson, Lars A., "Breastfeeding Stimulates the Infant Immune System," *Science & Medicine*, vol. 4, num. 6, November/ December, 1997.

Kirschmann, John D., Director, *Nutrition Almanac.* NY, NY: Nutrition Search Inc, 1990.

Kroh, Jacqueline, M.D., *The Whole Way to Natural Detoxification.* Point Roberts, WA: Hartley & Marks Publishers, Inc., 1996.

Lefkowitz SS and DL Lefkowitz, "Macrophage Candidicidal Activity of a Complete Glyconutritional Formulation versus Aloe Polymannose," *Proceedings of the Fisher Institute for Medical Research*, February, 1999.

Mindell, Earl, M.D., *Garlic The Miracle Nutrient.* New Canaan, CT: Keats Publishing, Inc., 1994.

Morris, Chris, N.D., *The True Nature of Healing.* Menlo Park, CA: The Publications Group, 1997.

Murray, Michael T., N.D., *Chronic Fatigue Syndrome.* Rocklin, CA: Prima Publishing, 1994.

Murray, Michael T., N.D., and Jade Beutler, R.R.T., R.C.P., *Understanding Fats & Oils.* Encinitas, CA: Progressive Health Publishing, 1996.

Pizzorno, Joseph, N.D., *Total Wellness.* Rocklin, CA: Prima Publishing, 1998.

The Promise, The Contemporary English Version. Nashville, TN: Thomas Nelson Publishers, 1995.

Ross, GP, MJ Polley and EM Rabellino, "Two Different Complement Receptors on Human Lymphocytes," *J Exp Med:* 1973, 138:798 – 818.

Samuels, Mike, M.D., and Nancy Samuels, *The Well Baby Book.* NY, NY: Simon & Schuster, 1991.

Schmidt, Michael A. D.C., C.C.N., *Childhood Ear Infections.* Berkeley, CA: North Atlantic Books, 1990.

Schmidt, Michael A., Lendon H. Smith and Keith W. Sehnert, *Beyond Antibiotics.* Berkeley, CA: North Atlantic Books, 1994.

See, Darryl, Ph.D., *Breakthrough Discoveries in Immune System Disorders.* Visua.Com: 1998.

See, Darryl, Ph.D., *Journal of the American Nutraceutical Association (JANA)*, Winter, 1999, vol. 2, no. 1.

Sehnert, Keith W., M.D., "The Garden Within — Acidophilus Candida Connection," Burlingame, CA: *Health World Magazine*, 1989.

"Special Report: Effect of Aloe Polymannose and Glyconutritionals on Candida," *Proceedings of the Fisher Institute for Medical Research:* February, 1999, vol. 1, no. 1.

Storkus, WJ and JR Dawson, "Target Structures Involved in Natural Killing (NK): Characteristics, Distribution and Candidate Molecules," *Critical Reviews in Immunology:* 1990, 10.

Tessler, Gordon S, Ph.D., *Breaking the Fat Barrier.* Raleigh, NC: Be Well Publications, 1993.

Townsley, Cheryl, *Cleansing Made Simple.* Littleton, CO: LFH Publishing, 1996.

Townsley, Cheryl, *Food Smart!* N, NY: Tarcher Putnam, 1998.

Townsley, Cheryl, *Kid Smart! Raising a Healthy Child.* Littleton, CO: LFH Publishing, 1996.

Zand, Janet, Lac, OMD, Rachel Walton, R.N., Bob Rountree, M.D., *Smart Medicine for a Healthier Child.* Garden City Park, NY: Avery Publishing Group, 1994.

INDEX

♦♦♦

gluten, 102
glyco, 24
glyconutirents, 28, 38, 43, 7987, 94, 107-108
glycoproteins, 24
grains, 90
granola, 123
granola-like breakfast, 123
granulocytes, 19, 22
green powder, 87, 94, 122
green produce, 15
grief, 50
groin, 26
guacamole dip, 127
guilt, 50, 80

H
hair loss, 30
hatred, 50
headaches, 50, 60
healing crisis, 27
heart disease, 47
heartburn, 54, 60, 72
hemorrhoids, 55
hepatocytes, 26
herbal cleanse, 85, 87
herbal liver cleanse, 84
herbs, 77
Heritage Store, 118
hives, 56
homeopathics, 40
honey, 71
hope, 63
Horizon, 11
hormonal imbalances, 41
hormones, 23

hostility, 50
household cleaners, 118
humus, 128
hydrochloric acid, 34, 74
hydrogenated fats, 14
hyperactivity, 40
hypoglycemia, 46

I
IBS, 55
Ig, 28-29
IgA, 28-29
IgE, 28-29
IgG, 28-29
IgM, 28-29
immune structure, 19
immune symptoms, 56
immune system, 87
immunoglobins, 28
impotence, 59
indigestion, 54, 60
infertility, 34, 41
inflammatory diseases, 44
inflexibility, 50
insect venom, 34
insecticides, 57
insecurity, 51
insulin imbalances, 45
interferons, 28
interleukins, 28
intestinal cramps, 54
intestinal gas, 54, 60
intestines, 26
iritation, 51
irritability, 60
irritable bowel syndrome, 55

Lifestyle for Health Order Form

Books

Discovering Wholeness, Townsley	26.95
Food Smart!, Townsley	13.00
Kid Smart!, Townsley	15.00
Cleansing Made Simple, Townsley	10.00
Candida Simple, Townsley	12.00
Return to Paradise, Townsley	10.00
Healthy Habits, Frähm	13.00

Cookbooks

Lifestyle for Health Cookbook, Townsley	26.00
Meals in 30 Minutes, Townsley	15.00
Candida Control Cookbook, Burton	14.00
Stevia Sweet Recipes, Goettemoeller	13.95

Audio Education

Too Stressed to Be Blessed (4 tapes)	25.00
Raging Hormones (4 tapes)	25.00
Healthy Kids – Beating ADD (2 tapes)	15.00
Supplements – A Systems Approach (1 tape)	5.00
Health & Supplements on a Budget (1 tape)	5.00
Optimal Health Video	25.00
Skin Brushing the Gaither Way	30.00

Supplements

YeastMAX – Candida Cleanse	30.00
ParaMAX – Parasite Cleanse	30.00
CleanseMAX – Bowel and Organ Cleansing	25.00
Barlean's Flax Seed Oil – 16 oz.	12.50
Barlean's Flax Seed Oil – 32 oz.	24.50
Barlean's Flax Seek Oil Capsules – 100 count	7.50
Ultra Pro Chocolate Protein Powder – 2 lbs.	49.00
Naturade Vegetable Protein Powder – 16 oz.	16.00
Designer Protein, Vanilla – 12 oz.	17.00
Designer Protein, Vanilla – 2 lbs.	36.00

Supplements

Catalyst Multi-Vitamin & Mineral – 120 count	42.00
Trace Minerals Concentrace Mineral Drops – 4 oz.	13.50
Trace Minerals Calcium & Magnesium – 120 count	17.00
Unique E – 400 I.U. each – 90 count	23.00
PhytoBears – kid's phytonutrient supplement	19.50
Barlean's Greens – 9.3 oz. powder	31.00
ImmunoStart™ – colostrum, beta-1,3 / 1,6 glucans & lactoferrin	42.50
DSF – de-stress formula – 60 count	21.00
GlycoBears – children's multi-vitamin/mineral – 60 count chewables	22.00
Plus – wild yam/hormone support – 90 count	39.00
Natural Progesterone Cream	25.00
Natren Megadophilus – small intestine support	22.00
Natren Bifido – large intestine support	22.00
Kyo-dophilus – 90 count	19.00
N-Zime #10 – general digestive enzyme support – 90 count	17.00

*(Visit our web site and complete the enzyme questionnaire
to find the enzyme(s) best suited for you.)*

Enzyme Solutions #1 – #36 (____ indicate #)	17.00

(All Enzyme Solutions prices are the same except the following.)

Enzyme Solutions #17, #34 or #35 (____ indicate #)	30.00
Enzyme Solutions #33	40.00

Glyconutrients

Ambrotose Bulk Powder 100 grams – 8 month supply	125.00
Ambrotose Bulk Powder 50 grams – 4 month supply	69.00
Ambrotose Capsules 60 count	39.00

Other

Blood Type Self Test Kit	15.00
Skin Brush – natural bristle	8.00
Shower Filter	49.00
Shower Filter Replacement Cartridge	25.00
Half-Fold Rebounder ($18 shipping fee)	249.00
Urban Rebounding Exercise Video	25.00
Bring Your Body to Life Exercise Program	99.00

ORDER FORM

ITEM NAME	QTY.	PRICE	TOTAL
		Subtotal	
		Shipping & Handling — add 15% (maximum $6.00)	
		Tax (CO residents 3.8%)	
		Total	

For fastest service fax your credit card order to 303-794-1449
or order on our secure website at www.lifestyleforhealth.com

Charge to my ☐ VISA or ☐ MASTERCARD

Card # _____ Exp. Date _____

Authorization Signature _____

Name _____

Address _____

City _____ State _____ Zip _____

Day Phone (____) _____

Send check or money order to:
Lifestyle for Health
6520 S. Broadway
Littleton, CO 80121
303-794-4477

AUTHOR
✦✦✦

Cheryl Townsley, N.D. is the founder of Lifestyle for Health, a company dedicated to helping people restore their total health to its full God-given potential. Cheryl has been a keynote speaker for national seminars, conferences and trade associations. She has been featured on hundreds of national and international television and radio programs.

Cheryl is known for her insight and humor, evident as she provides practical strategies to restore health. All, from individuals to whole families, will find opportunity to step into health with hope and encouragement with Cheryl.

Since 1991, Cheryl has published nine books: *Food Smart!*, *Lifestyle for Health* cookbook, *Meals in 30 Minutes*, *Kid Smart!*, *Return to Paradise*, *Candida Made Simple*, *Cleansing Made Simpple*, *Discovering Wholeness* and *Healthy Giving*.

Cheryl resides in Denver, Colorado, with her husband, Forest, and their daughter, Anna.